REVERSE THERAPY

CHRONIC FATIGUE, FIBROMYALGIA AND RELATED DISORDERS

JOHN EATON

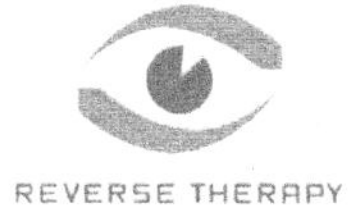

To Contact John Eaton:

Email: drjohneaton@gmail.com

Post: 4 Church St., Kintbury, Berkshire. RG17 9TR UK

Reverse Thinking Blog: www.reversethinking.co.uk

Reverse Therapy Site: www.reverse-therapy.com

In Memoriam

Milton Hyland Erickson

1901-1980

CONTENTS

ABOUT THE AUTHOR

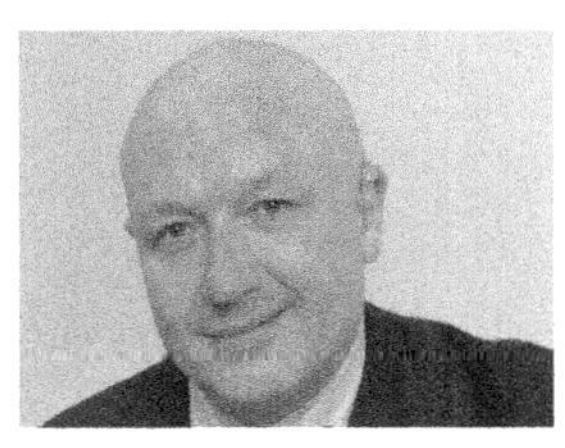

Dr John Eaton PhD has been practising since 1990 and is a registered psychotherapist with the United Kingdom Council for Psychotherapy. Between 1996 and 2002 he developed the ideas, principles and techniques that became Reverse Therapy. He gained his doctorate in Psychology from the University of Lancaster in 1998. He has written numerous books and articles on Reverse Therapy, psychotherapy, coaching and emotional intelligence.

He lives and works in Kintbury, Berkshire with his wife and family.

To Contact John:
www.reverse-therapy.com
drjohneaton@gmail.com

FOREWORD

A client of mine has just left me with renewed hope by the perspective that I shared with him on his Chronic Fatigue Syndrome. He realised he could now take the initiative and get well. So what had I shared? The perspectives that John has developed over years of clinical practice, and which he has generously captured in his latest book.

Reverse Therapy remarkably takes us through a journey that touches on autobiography, a portrait gallery of influential thinkers on the operation of the mind, his own clinical experience, and finally a practical guide to how the process works. The reader can dip into different sections. The earlier sections provide the foundations for the all-important second half.

The writing is clear, and the advice is explicit, but this underplays the understanding, the almost prophetic insights of the writer. It takes courage to go against received wisdom on Chronic Fatigue Syndrome,

Fibromyalgia and similar disorders. What is shared in the book is rooted in evidence; there is no requirement to sleep with your head aligned to magnetic north or adopt an idiosyncratic diet. Rather, this is evidence related wisdom from a man who has taken the time to step back from the battlefront, reflect and devise a different path. Of course, the critical factor is that it actually works!

The book provides tools not only for starting living again, but also tools for life's journey. I would suggest that whilst the book has an understandable focus on specific complaints, it should be mandatory reading for all of us who want improved emotional and physical health.

This is a book to be read by health-care professionals, counsellors, psychotherapists, psychiatrists and the afflicted themselves. For those who suffer, what is there to lose? Perhaps just months and years of confusion and misery.

Dr. Max Coates, London University (Institute of Education).

1

INTRODUCTION

Harriet's case (Part 1)

I first met Harriet when she came to my office, telling me she had been ill with Chronic Fatigue Syndrome (CFS) for seven years. She did not look well: drawn, haggard and weary. That was not surprising given her constant fatigue and pain, to mention but two symptoms. She was 33 but had been in so much pain over the past few years that she was now partly house-bound.

Although she had been diagnosed with CFS six years before, she thought the fatigue had been there on and off since she was a teenager. As she told me her life-story, some facts became apparent.

Harriet's parents separated when she was 12, and she lived with her mother and older sister. Her mother was a cold, hard woman who shouted at her whenever she did something wrong. Her sister was a few years older and attended another school, but they were never close. She always felt alone, and that life was too much for her, particularly school. She recalled her first menstrual period and being frightened by the blood (her mother had neglected to explain about puberty) and thinking she had some desperate illness, yet scared to tell anyone. When she confided in someone she thought was a friend, the other girls ridiculed her. That incident confirmed that it was best to keep her troubles to herself.

Although she was considered bright, she struggled with her GCSEs and 'A' Levels. She recalled feeling anxious much of the time that she would never get the grades her mother and her teachers expected (her sister had gone to Oxford to study Medicine and it was assumed Harriet would do the same). Whenever she had to write an essay, or revise for an exam, she would worry and lose sleep; whenever she got less than top marks, she would dread her mother berating her. In the end she 'only' got one top grade at A level, an outcome over which she experienced a lot of guilt, but she did get a place at a good university, studying law.

She felt just as lonely at university as she had at sixth form. She had few friends and was cripplingly shy. Nor did she find it easy to talk to her tutors when she struggled with course-work. The fatigue worsened and (thinking it was 'tiredness') she found it hard to get out of bed. She found it difficult to concentrate on her work, missed lectures, and took more time off sick. She went home for a few weeks but did not get well and felt worse after her mother told her to 'pull yourself together and get on with it'.

Through sheer persistence, and with some luck she achieved a second-class degree in law which, while not perfect, at least enabled her to get a job in a Solicitor's office as a trainee specialising in property law. She moved to London and started work. One of the other trainees at the office offered her a room in a shared house with two other women, with all of whom she made friends. Slowly life got better. For a while her fatigue and 'brain fog' went away entirely. After a year or so of this hard-working, but pleasant life she met a man to whom she was attracted, and began a relationship with him which lasted on-and-off for four years.

As she came closer to taking her professional exams, the symptoms resurfaced. This threw her into a panic as she was also managing a large portfolio of clients and she worried she would not qualify, or stay at the firm, if she became so ill that she could not work. But her worries only seemed to make the symptoms worse. None of the medical doctors she consulted seemed to know what was wrong with her. Nor did the many blood tests she underwent reveal anything amiss. One doctor offered her antidepressant drugs, but when she asked what good they might do the doctor shrugged and said there was nothing else he could offer. Harriet gained the distinct impression that this doctor thought that her illness was all in her head, a view her mother repeated with enthusiasm whenever she came to dinner. The idea that she was a malingering nuisance added still more to her isolation and fear, and still the symptoms worsened.

Her boyfriend, James, had always been an easy-going man but he, too, became impatient with her constant anxiety and panic, and with what he saw as the stop-start nature of her illness, in which one day she could go out with him, but the next spent in bed. By degrees he spent less and less time with her and rarely answered her calls. After one terrific row which followed his admission that he was dating other women, Harriet noticed a sharp, stabbing pain in her chest, and aching arms and legs. Shortly afterwards the relationship ended, but the pain did not go.

Fortunately, her employers were more understanding, and allowed her to work part time from home. They also gave her generous leave arrangements which enabled her, eventually and after many delays, to complete her exams and qualify as a solicitor. Even so, she believed that taking time off from work damaged her career chances, and that her employers secretly believed she was incapable. So she strove to work as hard as she could and to rest in between her spells of work. Before long she had given up going out, seeing friends or pursuing leisure interests, and her life consisted solely of work and rest. Just before she came to see me she was caught in what seemed like a never-ending cycle of stress from a failed relationship, her Mother's criticisms, the pressure of work, her worries over her future prospects, and the unrelenting symptoms of pain, fatigue, and brain fog, amongst others.

It may please the reader to learn that Harriet got well with the aid of Reverse Therapy. However, I will describe how she achieved her recovery in the last chapter of this book, once I have finished explaining how Reverse Therapy actually works.

(Note: names and some circumstances for all clients mentioned in this book have been changed to preserve anonymity).

The epidemics of chronic fatigue and fibromyalgia

I mention Harriet's case now as it is a sadly representative example of the suffering and isolation that too often comes with medically unexplained illness. It is also a good example of the cases we regularly see in Reverse Therapy.

Nor are such cases uncommon. A recent survey by the Centre for Disease Control and Prevention (CDC) in the USA estimated that the prevalence rate for Chronic Fatigue Syndrome is between 0.25% and 0.4% of the general population (I believe this figure may be an underestimate). If this estimate is correct, then there will be between 160,000 and 250,000 sufferers in the United Kingdom, and between 0.8 million and 1.3 million sufferers in the United States.

Turning to medically unexplained pain conditions, the figure for these conditions is even higher and, according to some sources, they are amongst the fastest growing illnesses in the USA. The CDC estimates that the prevalence rate for Fibromyalgia Syndrome (the most common medically unexplained pain disorder) is around 2%

which, if true, would suggest that there are 6.4 million sufferers in the United States alone.

Reverse Therapy was developed by me since 1996 in order to explain the origins and physical source of these conditions, and their solution. Along with Chronic Fatigue Syndrome and Fibromyalgia we have Burnout Syndrome, Tension Headaches, Irritable Bowel Syndrome, Colitis, and Tension Myositis. Additionally, there are the Auto-Immune diseases such as Rheumatoid Arthritis and Systemic Lupus, which are addressed by both non-medical and medical approaches.

Ignorance of, and misunderstandings about, these conditions seem to me to be widespread, and it is another purpose of this book to dispel these. Many people, like Harriet, find their suffering compounded by the wrong advice given to them by their consultants, the apparent lack of a cure, rejection by the people around them, and the isolation and fear that comes with having an illness with no clear-cut medical criteria for diagnosis or resolution.

The notion that symptoms of Chronic Fatigue Syndrome and Fibromyalgia are 'all in the mind' is one example of ignorance. As we shall see, this is very far from being the case. The symptoms are in fact created by neurological and glandular changes in the body and are very real indeed! These changes are triggered by signals from the limbic system working through the HPA Axis and vagus Nerve under the overall direction of what I, following Candace Pert and other writers, call 'Bodymind'.

Towards a new type of therapy

One important theme of this book – in fact it is a key to understanding Reverse Therapy – is that in considering the origin of these conditions we reverse the priority given to thinking mind in our culture, and focus our attention on bodymind – the source of feelings, emotions, intuitions and our deeply felt decisions. For it is also the source of the disorders described in this book. When the body becomes distressed by life events, it triggers a string of neurological changes which results in the symptoms of Chronic Fatigue and related disorders. Understanding how this happens can provide us with clues for understanding and treating the epidemic of medically unexplained illnesses we are now seeing in the world today.

Reverse Therapy is part of the new, worldwide movement towards therapies that work with bodymind. It is a healing process which reverses symptoms by understanding why the body created them. It is based on discoveries in neuroscience which have (mostly) been taking place in the United States over the past 30 years.

Some of these discoveries relate to:

- The workings of the limbic system (also known as the Emotional Brain)
- The link between emotions and health
- The connections between the brain, the endocrine system, the immune system, and the nervous system

- How the body uses cellular memories to store information about emotional threats
- How bodymind creates emotions using hormones, nerve signals, and neuropeptides
- The stress-disease connection
- The alarm mechanisms which lead to symptom formation.
- The causes of non-specific illnesses such as Chronic Fatigue Syndrome and Fibromyalgia

In this book I explain how medically unexplained illnesses are not psychosomatic, but are created through interactions between the environment, the mind, the emotions, the brain, the endocrine system and the nervous system. My explanation is not complete, as much research has still to be carried out on the precise nature of these interconnections. But a holistic theory of this kind - which will eventually lead to a genuine solution for these illnesses - is sorely overdue. Reverse Therapy is a prototype for such a cure.

Reverse Therapy is a simple process in which people learn to listen to the body and understand the deeper reasons for how the body gets distressed, and why symptoms are the natural result. Tied to this is the perception that the symptoms themselves are warning signals which provide clues to a solution. This process of enlightenment goes side-by-side with dropping the many wrong and confused ideas people have been given about the relationship between environmental stress, unresolved emotions, unhealthy thinking patterns, and breakdowns in physical health.

I have been learning, developing and experimenting with the ideas in this book since 1996. I would like to clarify that few of the ingredients that go to make up Reverse Therapy are new, although the synthesis is, and the unique step-by-step treatment process.

The theoretical basis for Reverse Therapy comes largely from the advances in neuroscience which have taken place over the past twenty-five years. Some eminent names here include Candace Pert, Joseph LeDoux, Anthony Damasio, Esther Sternberg, Richard Davidson, Sharon Begley, Gabor Maté, and George Porges.

Naturally, I have learnt the most from my clients – who, along the way, have taught me how to improve delivery of Reverse Therapy. I have been fortunate in learning, also, from many outstanding teachers. These include Bill O'Hanlon, Stephen Gilligan, Ernest Rossi, Richard Bandler and, standing behind us all, Milton Erickson. I have also learnt a great deal from the work of Wilhelm Reich, Fritz Perls and Eugene Gendlin. To all these men and women, I owe a debt of thanks.

Final note. This book first appeared in 2017, based on an earlier version published in 2005. This is the second edition, republished in 2021, which has been revised and updated.

2

THE ORIGINS OF REVERSE THERAPY

My early experiences

Reverse Therapy is continually evolving. But when I came to give this approach a name in 2002 it had, by then, emerged from four unique sources:

- My own troubled experiences as a young man
- What I learnt in therapy
- What I learnt from other therapists
- Personal exposure to medically unexplained illnesses

I will describe all these elements in their proper place.

I begin with an experience which first brought home to me the experience of bodily distress. This experience, which at the time I considered a breakdown, was one of the most disturbing of my entire life. It was also profoundly educational.

I was then in the third year of employment as a printer's apprentice in 1974 and I was eighteen years old. I had been more or less thrown out of my grammar school at fifteen for misbehaviour and my father, from the old-fashioned working-class thought it better anyway that I gave up education and learned a trade. Glad to be away from the hated school, I readily agreed. The first year was fine, but then I awoke to the fact that I found the work boring. Setting up, and proof-reading type, and then clearing it all away again soon became monotonous. Nor did I like the mean-minded attitude of the journeymen around me, and their distaste for ideals. In fact, I learnt that most printers, although they physically create books and magazines, have little interest in reading anything themselves, aside from tabloid newspapers. They themselves printed journals every working day, but had little interest in what they actually meant.

Although I loathed the 'education' I had received at the grammar school, I was seriously interested in ideas. I dreamed of studying philosophy, or depth psychology at university, and then becoming a writer. But I came from a working-class family in South London in which people did not go to such places. Strangely, I had a few friends (from the grammar school) who went to University, but few of them were really interested in ideas. Their main pre-occupations seemed to be dope-smoking, LSD, psychedelic music and sex. All this (plus the fact that I wasn't getting much sex) left me thinking I was some kind of freak, doomed to live in a dream-world which had little connection with the tedious reality of everyday life. As I grew more and more alienated, I became more and more depressed.

At that time, an apprentice signed 'Articles' which bound him to the employer for six years. I could only be released from them with the agreement of the employer at a request from my father. On seeking my father's help, he flatly refused to intercede. I wanted to go back to college, which he saw as a waste of time and would mean giving up the promise of a solid trade. Defying him would mean leaving home and working in another grim factory, so no escape there. Rather like Gordon Comstock in George Orwell's *Keep the Aspidistra Flying*, I settled down to this hateful existence and wrote poems about it in my spare time.

One Monday, at precisely 11.50 a.m., while I was staring at the big clock that hung over the composing room, I experienced a massive panic attack. Something alien was rising through my body with tremendous force. I couldn't breathe and my heart was beating so fast I thought I might die. My body would not stop shaking and the sweat poured off me. The entire episode could not have lasted over two minutes, yet it seemed to go on for an eternity. I was still staring at the clock and noticed that, weirdly, the hands did not seem to move. The sheer strangeness of it all made me think I might go mad.

To avoid the suspicion that I was going insane, I took steps to act as if everything was 'normal' (I was hidden out of sight of most people anyway, behind my composing desk). After a while the panic faded away and eventually I went home and tried to forget about it. However, this proved to be only the start. Although I did

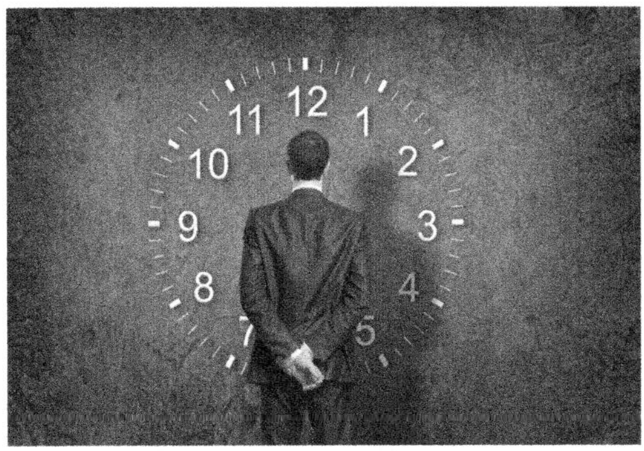

The feeling that time has stopped is, in fact, quite common during traumatic experiences.

not want to think about what was happening to me, my body had other ideas.

From then on, on every day of the week while at work, the seizure returned at precisely 11.50 am. As the clock ticked on through the morning, I prepared myself for the attack that was sure to come. The moment the first hand moved to '10' there would come an uprising in my torso, like a pressure cooker coming to the boil. Then the shaking would start. Then the rest of the symptoms would fire. I could not avoid them, or control them and could only wait for them to go. Eventually, after a week of this, the supervisor came over to me and asked if I was 'all right'. Realising my secret was out, I told him my dreadful story (I omitted the detail about the hands on the clock stopping at 11.50 am). To my surprise, he was sympathetic and told me to take a few days off and see a doctor.

I went to see my GP the next day. Dr Todd had treated me since I was a child and when he heard of my condition, he took the trouble to spend a half-hour with me (he was a very busy man yet held up his surgery for my sake). Explaining what a panic attack was, he told me it was typically the outcome after a long period of stress. He then told me about his experiences as a member of a bomber air crew during the war, when he was barely out of his teens. Almost nightly, he and the rest of the crew went through the risk of being shot at, blown up, set on fire, or bailing out to drown in the North Sea. He had seen many of his friends break down from stress or from trauma, as he had once himself. He explained that many of them carried on through a sense of duty to their country but, in this case, my duty was to myself. If I was unhappy, then it was important that I made the right decision to get my emotional health back. He told me he would not prescribe any drugs for me as they would not solve the real problem. He encouraged me to think over what it was I was really unhappy about and what I wanted to do about it, if not now then later.

Possibly, Dr Todd saved my life. Without his advice I might have ended up in an institution (this was the 1970s and mental health services were then limited to crude psychiatry), or in something worse. I confessed all to my parents This time my father accepted I was in a bad way and agreed to get me released from the articles. The next term I enrolled at college to study English and History and, after a few months in a new and more rewarding environment, the panic attacks gradually ceased.

I did not realise the significance of this experience until years later, after I got on the path that led to Reverse Therapy. It seemed to be one of those inexplicable and disturbing things the body might do when people were stressed. Yet I did not even understand what stress was.

Nor did I understand that bodymind had been attempting to communicate with me for some time before the panic attacks started, by sending me warning messages through frustration and fear, and a 'pressure-cooker' feeling of inner turmoil coming to the boil. Because I was too ignorant to recognise these feelings for what they were, because no one around me could help me deal with them, and because I was afraid of acting on my own, I suppressed them. But bodymind is stronger than we might think, and all that denial did was fuel the panic attacks. Only by taking my doctor's advice and acting on the needs that underpinned the original emotions could the panic be dispelled. Much time was to pass before I understood the subtle logic behind symptoms like these.

My experiences in therapy

I would like to have been able to write that, after my experiences with the clock-bound panic attacks, I grew up wiser and more emotionally intelligent. But I did not really understand my recovery and nor did I care to think much about it, so disturbing it had been. But when my marriage broke down some years later, I was again in emotional trouble.

In copy-cat fashion I was stuck in an unrewarding job (I have noticed this again and again in my later work as a therapist – conditioning leads to people 'always crashing in the same car', repeating the same mistakes again and again, until they learn otherwise). After university, and a brief stab at writing novels and poems, I went into financial services for no better reason than that banks paid well and jobs there carried some prestige (or so I thought). Although I enjoyed managing and developing teams of people, I detested office politics. I also disliked the cynicism and frivolity of the banking world. I was bored and drinking heavily, bad-tempered at home. My wife, Yvonne, put up with this for a while but soon grew tired of it as she herself was having problems at work and was going through a crisis of her own. She moved out of our home in Berkshire and went to stay in London, saying that it would be better for both of us if we separated. Unwilling to lose her, I agreed to see a psychotherapist together with her. However, it was quickly realised that it would be better for me to work with the therapist on my own.

I knew nothing of how therapy worked in practice and had assumed that, after a few confessionals, I could resume my marriage and go back to the way things were before. Fortunately, Nigel, my therapist, had other ideas. He pointed to my poor emotional intelligence, my frequent rages, my underlying depression, my unresolved dissatisfaction with life, and my relationship problems, and urged me to look deeper.

Nigel himself always appeared composed and gave me the impression that my weaknesses, while I should discard them, were human-all-too-human and not unique to me: a matter for sorrow and regret rather than blame. In my subsequent career as a therapist, I have tried to reproduce this approach to human frailty as well as I can, not always with success. Interestingly, Nigel was not primarily interested in psychotherapy. He was a mystic who ran training groups in Sufism. I have noticed throughout my career that people who are good at therapy tend not to be therapists by choice, and many of them have little formal training. There may be a moral here somewhere.

Nigel told me that my irritability, my depression and my boredom with life resulted from dishonesty with myself and with others, with a loss of connection with my emotions and my subsequent inability to articulate them, or to resolve them. Much of our work together revolved around this. I wanted to achieve the same air of serenity, and the feeling of being comfortable inside my skin that Nigel had.

In therapy, good questions can make the difference between success and failure. Nigel was an adept at asking the right questions at the right time. His questions, partly based on Socratic method, forced me to re-think my assumptions about things I had always taken for granted.

For example, I remember telling him once that I couldn't help my low moods, they 'just happened' (I often got depressed when I was younger and had been told by my mother it was 'the family curse', carrying the implication that there was little I could do about it). Immediately, Nigel asked:

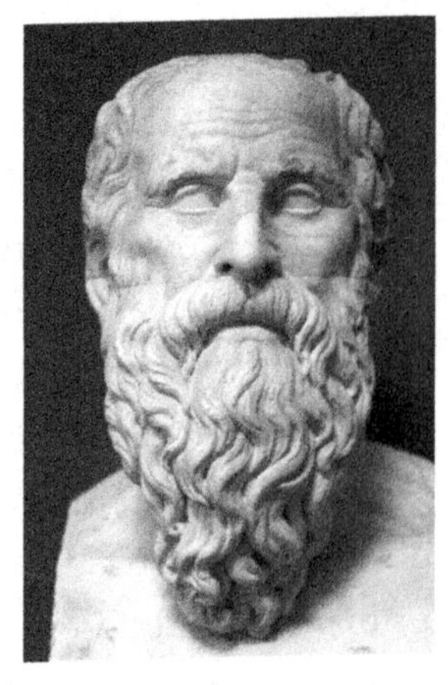

Socrates 469-399 BC employed a question-and-answer technique which forced his to define their terms, eventually realising that their views were inadequate. He said of himself 'I know that I am wise because I know that I know nothing.'

"Yes, and when they are about to happen, how do you know that is the case?"

It took a long time for me to see the answer and when I did, I realised that I always 'knew' when my low moods were about to happen. Usually, I would feel restless and on edge for hours or even days at a time. Without knowing it, my body was sending me subtle signals that something was up and that I was out of touch with my real wishes. When the discomfort became too great, my emotions were automatically 'de-pressed' by me, leaving me feeling numb and empty and even more out of touch with myself. This led to countless problems in relationships, and in my finding my proper path in life. Side by side with this realisation I saw that there was a subtle conditioning process that had been going on throughout my life up to that point. Somehow I had learned - from other people - to de-press emotions and fall into depression, and there was a pattern to it. And the implication was that, if I had learnt that pattern, then I could unlearn it.

Another question, repeated several times, related to the purpose of my reactions, as opposed to my delusions about them. For example, one day I described an episode in which I was at a party and the room crowded with noisy, 'up-and-coming' types amongst whom I felt awkward and shy. Asked to explore and express the feeling that came with my 'shyness' I realised I had not felt shy at all, but repelled by the some of the people there, and I simply wished not to talk. The child in me did not want to join in the barnyard pecking order (which reminded me of the school) because to do so would have ended with my pretending to be someone I was not. What I had interpreted as a lack of self-assurance was, instead, the reverse: a much deeper feeling of the kind only children (or child-like adults) can understand.

Other questions would have the effect of opening up a fresh way of seeing something, and in those moments I would have the feeling that I had dropped burdens I had been carrying for years. Typically, these questions focused on the rules and injunctions I carried around in my head – the 'must do this' and 'have to do that' or 'got to do it this way' judgments I took for granted. For example, I had for a long time assumed that I had to be in control of life (possibly a result of my earlier brush with insanity). Now I saw how much unnecessary distress this control-freakery had caused to me and to others. I learnt that most of these rules were complete exaggerations or just plain nonsense that I had taken over from other people! Learning to make up my own (flexible) rules and avoid the word 'must' were the keys to that discovery.

By the time I had ended therapy (it took a year) I knew one thing: I wanted to do the things Nigel made look so easy. I wanted to learn enough about human beings so that I, too, could know exactly where to look for the root of their disorder. And then I would know which questions to ask! I did not know then that a skill like this takes years to develop and I am still learning as I write.

A year after leaving therapy, I left financial services and retrained as a psychotherapist. Over the years I qualified in Counselling, Hypnotherapy, Rational-Emotive Therapy, Stress Management and Brief Solution-focused Therapy, but the approach that most fascinated me was Milton Erickson's Strategic Therapy. I was struck by the simplicity and strangeness of his work, and by its emotional depth.

What I learnt from Erickson and Rossi

Milton Erickson was an American psychiatrist who did his best work from the 1940s to the 1970s. While most psychiatrists at that time used drugs, surgery, electroshock techniques, and psychoanalysis to treat their patients Erickson employed a strategic approach based on his interpretation of what his patient's unconscious mind wanted to do next. He rejected the idea that the unconscious mind was neurotic and stuck in the past, insisting that it was an active, problem-solving intelligence acting in the present. All that the physician had to do was establish what its purposes were.

Consider these cases:

A man with chronic headaches who prided himself on his honesty was cured by advising him that his headaches were there because he was being dishonest about his difficulties with his family, and it was time he did something about it. The headaches faded after he told his wife it was time she disciplined the children more.

A woman with depression, which followed a long history of abuse and rejection from her parents, was taught to reconnect to her anger over her treatment by them, accept her 'shocking' emotions, and also her right to build a life on her own terms, away from her parents.

A woman with digestive problems was cured after Erickson heard her say that she couldn't 'stomach' her bullying sister. Her issue cleared up after she told her sister, under instructions from Erickson, to stop calling her up on the phone every day with unwanted 'advice'.

A woman with asthma wanted to find out why it was she only ever had asthma during the winter months. Erickson had noted earlier that she received threatening letters from her father every winter, accusing her of stealing property he claimed was due to him from her mother's will. Under hypnosis she made the connection between the asthma attacks and the letters from her father for herself. The asthma attacks ceased after she hired a lawyer to write a letter to her father.

I picked these specific examples, which all relate to unwanted symptoms of one kind or another, because they illustrate a principle I learnt from Erickson and which is a key part of the Reverse Therapy approach. That is the importance of understanding what symptoms are doing in our lives before we try to change them, much less resist them. Making a connection between symptoms and the situations that triggered them led first to emotional insight, then to acceptance of the purpose of the symptoms, and then on to uncovering the actions required.

There is much more to Erickson's work than this, but I am only referring to the elements which bear directly on Reverse Therapy and the underlying theme of this book.

Another aspect of Erickson's work was his interest in unconscious communication. Erickson believed in the unconscious mind – I no longer do so because I believe that most of what we think of as the 'Unconscious Mind' is actually bodymind intelligence. However that may be, Erickson thought that the Unconscious had important reasons for producing symptoms – reasons that had to do with protecting the self from harm.

For example, he once worked with a woman with psoriasis. This is a disabling skin condition that causes severe itching, scaling and rashes. The woman had a troubled life with many stressors, mostly involving family conflict. Erickson listened to her stories for a while before asking her to roll up her sleeve so that he could look at her rash. Then he observed, offhand, that she 'had a lot of emotion but only a little psoriasis'. The woman was so angry with what she imagined were Erickson's belittling remarks, she got up and left. A week later she called to tell Erickson that she had been furious with him, and with her family, but the rash was fading away and she wanted to know why.

Notice that in walking out of his office, the patient was already falling into line with what Erickson had suggested ('... you have a lot of emotions...') and is setting herself up for the solution. The more emotions she noticed, the less her unconscious mind - her body - was forced to produce symptoms to tell her it was time she did something about them. Walking out on Erickson was one way she acted on that message; telling people in her family a few home truths was another. In that way the original emotions were released, and so was the distress that contributed to her skin problem.

Erickson's work has been extremely influential since he died in 1980, and many people who studied with him have established novel forms of therapy themselves. Reverse Therapy owes much to Erickson, in particular the insight that some symptoms have an unconscious meaning and purpose, and that healing comes about when we uncover that purpose.

One of Erickson's pupils – and co-writer of several books with Erickson – was Dr Ernest Rossi who made some further innovations in what he called '*Psychobiology*' (the study of mind-body communication) and in the development of new treatment approaches to the symptomatic states we are discussing. In his ground-breaking work

'The Psychobiology of Mind-Body Healing' Dr Rossi explains that the body registers significant learning experiences and stores the information away in the Emotional brain, and elsewhere in the body, as a cellular memory.

For example, when you learnt to ride a bike, the first few weeks were most likely painful. Multi-tasking the steering, balance, pedalling and braking meant frequent stops and starts, and quite a lot of falls. Eventually, your body 'got it' and, from that point on, cycling became a pleasure rather than an ordeal. The 'muscle memory' was available to you whenever you re-mounted the bike.

In the same way, the body stores memories about emotional learning. And, as we shall see later in the book, it stores away alarm reactions which result in symptomatic states.

Therapy can help people free themselves from symptoms when we tap into the cellular memory (Rossi calls this 'state-dependent memory') used by the unconscious mind (or body) to create warning signals about situations. Rossi uses a semi-hypnotic process to do this in which the client senses changes in the body (a hand movement, for example, or rising sensations in the chest) which contain unconscious communications of various kinds and allows them to be heard. In pursuing similar objectives in Reverse Therapy, we have established that hypnosis is not required in order to assist clients to make those connections.

When we find out what the emotional body has learned about these situations, and why they are a problem, we can help clients learn how to do something different. As they overcome the difficulty, bodymind picks up that there is no longer a problem and de-activates the cellular memory. When that happens, symptoms can disappear.

A direct experience of bodily distress

While I was trying to understand the work of Erickson and Rossi, and apply their lessons in clinical practice, my wife Yvonne developed a serious, life-threatening illness in 1996. In fact symptoms, in the form of mysterious viral complaints and gut disorders, had developed the year before. Those never entirely went away and, before long others came along too. Her toes, fingers and nose became inflamed, she was in constant nerve pain and, by degrees her feet, hands and the left side of her face became paralysed. After breaking down on Bonfire Night during a family party, she was rushed to hospital and diagnosed with neuro-sarcoidosis. In this form it is an extremely rare disease, difficult to treat and sometimes fatal. It is one of the auto-immune diseases.

An auto-immune condition refers to a breakdown in the immune system (our defence against infection) in such a way that it goes into overdrive, and its killer cells attack the body's healthy cells. Multiple Sclerosis is a well known example. Somehow, the immune system has learnt to view the cells it is protecting as a threat. In Yvonne's case her immune system was attacking the nerve cells in her feet, hands and face. When the cells are attacked, deposits (sarcoids) are left behind which gradually pile up and paralyse the cells. The usual treatment, then as now, is a course of steroids in high dosages which suppress the immune system altogether.

The causes of auto-immune diseases are still obscure, but it has become increasingly clear that emotional factors play a part in the build-up to illness. This was certainly true in Yvonne's case. Within 18 months she had lost both Grandmothers through death and underwent a horrific experience of work-place bullying at an American bank. We had also suffered a large financial loss which wiped out most of our savings when an investment went wrong. At the same time she was also coping with the challenges that came with raising our two young children, who were then six and four years old. I recall at that she did not complain, but seemed unnaturally despondent, although her burdens were huge.

Although I wanted to help Yvonne as much as I could, and wondered whether there was a therapy that might address her illness, there was little I could do except offer hypnosis for her nerve pain. But what emerged from Yvonne's experience was something from which she and I learned a great deal.

Once the condition stabilised, residual symptoms remained: muscle weakness, tiredness, pain, itching and sleep disturbance. Observation showed that the symptoms varied over a cycle lasting a few weeks. They would be easiest when she had plenty of quiet time with friends and family, harder when things were over-wrought at work. Reduced if she felt that she was on top of things;

worsened if she was under the cosh. From this it became clear that her emotional state was closely linked to her symptomatic state. This suggested that her immune system returned to something more like normal function when she was addressing problems at work, or restoring the work/life balance.

Using this clue, Yvonne looked harder at her difficulties with the bank. Effectively, her employers were trying to drive her away while pretending that they had her welfare at heart. She suffered particularly from the attentions of a manager who could best be described as a vindictive bully. In one encounter, while under attack for not meeting some impossible target, Yvonne stood up to her and told her what she thought of her 'management skills'. But this was only a partial solution, as it did not stop the intrigues from this woman and the other managers there. It merely made them more cautious with their schemes.

In time the solution was provided by changed circumstances. Yvonne was hospitalised for six weeks after the Bonfire Night collapse. She was on sick leave for four months after that. During this convalescence she received another job offer from a firm that had heard of her achievements and was keen to have her. She resigned from the toxic employer and moved to the new one on her recovery. There she was well-treated and began to enjoy work again. Meanwhile, my practice was growing larger and our financial difficulties faded away. Before too long the sarcoidosis had gone. It has returned slightly three or four times in the last twenty-five years, and the first sign is always a slight reddening of the nose. Each time Yvonne notices that particular symptom she knows that some remedial work is due.

The last piece in the jigsaw

As my practice developed, I came to see more and more cases in which puzzling and unexplained symptoms seemed to emerge from a period of emotional distress. Irritable bowel syndrome, skin complaints and unexplained headaches were among the most common. It seemed to me that the symptoms of anxiety and depression, to name the two most common mental health disorders, had a similar root, although I could not explain how.

At that time (late 1990s) I was still following Erickson and Rossi's lead: using hypnosis to explore what might lie behind the symptoms and help my clients understand their purpose. However, most of this work was hit-and-miss; sometimes successful and sometimes not. I still did not understand the mechanisms through which the body translates life problems and unsatisfied emotions into the symptoms of physical illness. Nor did I have a clear-cut way of 'talking' to the body, as the fallacy of the 'Unconscious Mind' still misled me.

An early case

A case that came my way revealed some clues. Peter was a successful solicitor who had suffered from irritable bowel syndrome for nine years. The symptoms were bloating, abdominal pain, diarrhoea and nausea. Peter knew vaguely that his condition became worse if he experienced worries over his family, or if he over-worked.

I advised him that his symptoms were the complex result of interactions between his mind, his body, his emotions and the environment. When he assented to this a trance state was induced and I suggested that the uncomfortable sensations in his abdomen contained an important message about his problem and soon he would know more about it. I asked him to remember a time when the symptoms were strong and pay attention to any associated feelings, images and thoughts that came up that would contain clues to 'the message'. After a while, a surprised look came over his face, but I left him in peace to 'digest' the message.

When he came around, he commented that an image of a gag had come up and he clearly got the idea that his symptoms appeared when he felt compelled to take on more burdens than he could bear, and that he did not have the right to refuse. His willingness to accept such demands came from his perfectionistic belief that he should work harder and harder in order to be successful - and that entailed sacrifice - even at the expense of his health. After that we worked on distinguishing between sustainable work and the unsustainable variety; on saying 'No' to excessive demands on his time; and on setting boundaries between work and private life.

Satisfied that he now had some new strategies that would help him deal with the problem, he went 'back inside' and 'asked' his symptom-state if it was happy with these newfound solutions. By way of an answer, his discomfort subsided. His IBS problem gradually cleared up as he became more disciplined in managing his work-load, and handling demands from other people. Soon, he was largely free of symptoms.

There were two things I learned indirectly from this case. One was that in investigating the source of the symptom, my client was really communicating to his body rather than to his unconscious mind. The second followed logically from the first: that it was unnecessary to use hypnosis to understand the symptom-message. In fact, trance-work can get in the way. For every two clients who found hypnosis easy to do and helpful in establishing communication with the body, there was one who did not. Some clients would be so intent on listening to my suggestions, and working up a trance state, they had little attention left over for working through the symptom. A more direct approach also meant that clients could learn to do it for themselves without my help.

In the Focusing approach pioneered by Eugene Gendlin clients work directly with the body, tune into uncomfortable feelings, and relay a series of questions to the problematic state in order to understand it better.

For example:

- 'What are you trying to tell me?'
- What do you do for me?'
- 'What are you trying to protect me from?'

- 'What can I learn from you?'

- 'What do you want me to do?'

I adapted this approach to the exploration of simple symptomatic states. For example, a felt tension in the jaw, throat, or chest that comes up whenever the individual is in conflict with other people. They then go through a process of simply 'asking' the symptom state (or the 'cellular memory' which lies behind it) what they should do next.

Answers might include:

- I am trying to tell you not to walk away from conflict

- I am trying to protect you from disrespect

- I am trying to teach you to be more honest about your feelings

- I want you to practice fresh ways to assert yourself

With more complex illnesses, however, this direct approach would not work. It would have been impossible to 'ask' Yvonne's sarcoids what they wanted. Similarly, it would be difficult to establish what an inflammation of the colon or an eczema rash that had been there for months what it was messaging right now – given that it was a reaction to events that had happened some time before. It was likely that mistakes the client had made before the symptoms appeared were still being made in the present. But how to ask bodymind for the right answers?

In Reverse therapy, as we have developed it now, we work in a more indirect way. We teach the client how to sense their body in different ways: feelings, sensations and emotions until this becomes an automatic skill. Exploring the meaning of symptoms by taking them back to life events in which the symptoms first appeared and looking at the pressures they were encountering. We ask them to recall the feelings, sensations, emotions and thoughts that were coming up then, getting a sense of what it was bodymind was trying to tell them through the symptoms *at that time*. Then we check what the body is seeking now.

The key here is to connect to bodymind during a period of distress which occurred just before onset of the symptoms when dealing with chronic, long-term symptoms, such as an irritable bowel, and to a moment of distress which occurred just before an increase in short-term symptoms such as pain and fatigue. To put it another way, we connect to the feelings and emotions behind the symptoms rather than to the symptoms themselves. Naturally, this may take some trial and error in practice.

It is important to understand that Reverse Therapy does not just analyse the cause of the symptom. For example, the answer to the question Why is this symptom there? might be: 'Because I am scared of people'. But the answer to the question: What is my body encouraging me to do about this?, might be: 'I want you to practice speaking to people you can trust about your problems'. Analysis alone is not enough; enlightenment about the body's purposes is the proper goal. In the last resort, bodymind requires action to resolve the problem so that it doesn't need to trigger the alarm mechanisms which follow on from distress.

One difference between Reverse Therapy and medical approaches is that in the latter the idea is to get rid of the symptoms of Chronic Fatigue Syndrome as quickly as possible. We treat symptoms as helpful messages that need to be understood first before they can go away – and they will certainly not depart until the client has learned to abide by their advice. The final difference is that we teach our clients how body intelligence actually works through the Emotional Brain and the HPA Axis to create the symptoms. I will say more about this in later chapters, but the key point is that knowing what is happening in the body when symptoms come up dispels anxiety. It also creates a space in which the symptoms can be accepted and understood.

Key points in this Chapter

- Reverse Therapy is based on the insight that many symptomatic states have an unconscious purpose
- Milton Erickson's *Strategic Therapy* addresses these purposes on the assumption that the Unconscious Mind is a problem-solving intelligence
- Ernest Rossi shows that some unconscious purposes are linked to cellular memories of past experiences

- Reverse Therapy substitutes 'Bodymind' for the 'Unconscious' Mind
- Eugene Gendlin's Focusing approach uses questions to access unconscious/bodymind issues
- Reverse Therapy addresses Chronic Fatigue Syndrome, Fibromyalgia and related disorders, by uncovering the underlying message behind the symptom

3

ABOUT BODYMIND

How bodymind works

The term 'Bodymind' refers to the intelligence of the body which, in this book, we contrast with mental intelligence. Whereas we think consciously in terms of words, concepts, images and visual memories and so forth, the body 'thinks' in terms of cellular communication: rapid transfers of information between cells in the eyes, ears, brain, the nervous system, the heart, the gut, skin and immune system, to name just a few sites. In order to understand how conditions such as Chronic Fatigue Syndrome arise, we need to understand how the body 'thinks' and what it is seeking to communicate through the symptoms. Also, to understand how the body, despite its deep intelligence, becomes distressed.

Since Plato in the 4th Century BC, western culture has marginalised the body, and idolised thinking mind, all the way up to Descartes in the 17th century, and beyond.

Later on in this book I will show that human beings are not nearly as rational as they think they are, but in this chapter I invite you to deepen your appreciation of the intelligence of the body. At the emotional level, it is far more profound than mental intelligence could ever be. Following it is not only the way to health but also the path to insight and fulfilment.

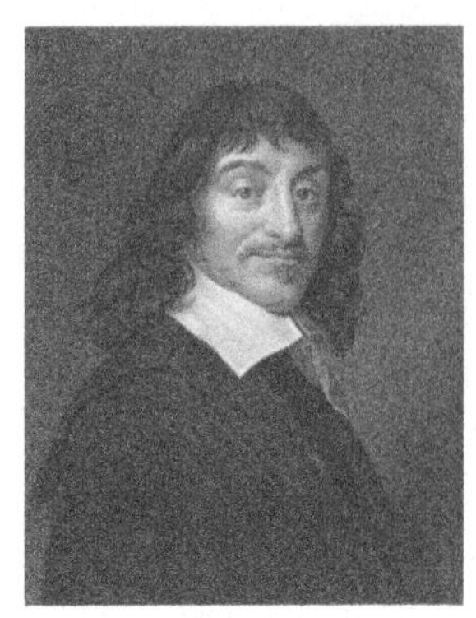

Rene Descartes 1596-1650 argued that thoughts in the conscious mind were the source of all reliable knowledge. His phrase 'Cogito Ergo Sum' (I think therefore I am) implies that they are all we can know for sure.

Considered closely, bodymind is miraculous in its complexity. There are around 37 trillion cells in the body, but each cell can have up to 10,000 connections to other cells (transmitting information in tenths of a second), forming neural networks which can make sophisticated, quick-fire decisions in a few seconds. Those decisions include:

- Tissue renewal and repair
- Metabolism and cell growth
- Temperature control
- Co-ordination of movement
- Digestion and excretion
- Sexual drives and reproduction

- Resisting infection
- Energy & the rest-activity cycle
- Arousal and attention
- Processing sensory information
- Emotional signalling
- Thought processes

The primary purpose of bodymind is survival, both of the individual and of the species, although personal survival depends partly on successful adaptation to changing environments, and partly on the satisfaction of instincts, drives and emotions. If individuals do not cope with threat and do not satisfy their drives towards security, love and satisfying work, amongst other desires, then they are less likely to reproduce, and the survival of the species will remain in question.

We can see some of these drives working through Abraham Maslow's Hierarchy of Needs.

In the diagram below we can see bodymind purposes working up the scale to fit the person for life. It preserves first basic physical health, then the reduction of threat, then the formation of relationships (personal and communal). Following on from that we have achievement, recognition, and respect from others. However, that is largely matter for the ego rather than for the self (more about that in the next chapter). But the last step is interesting, as it bears on long-term psychological health. Self-actualisation entails satisfaction from making the most of your opportunities, your talents, your interests and the things you love to do. It is a fact that cheerful people are healthier people and healthy people (barring accidents, disease and war) live longer.

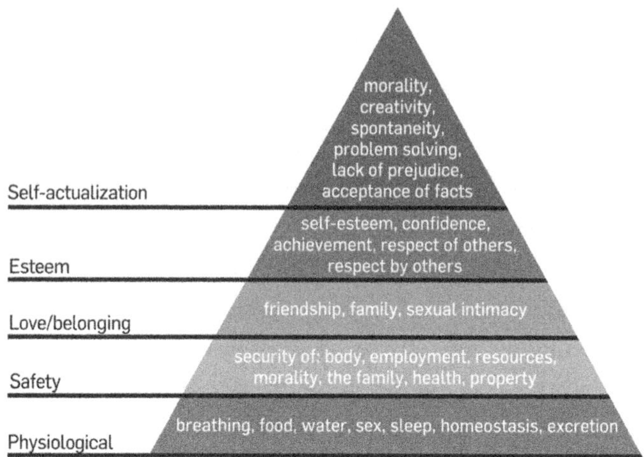

As we shall note later, the body uses emotions to guide us towards self-actualisation, thus preserving and expanding our existence.

One way to think about bodymind and its cellular networks is to liken it to a large city. Inside the city are ring-roads and streets; squares, parks and shopping malls; apartments, houses and offices; and command centres distributed throughout the city: town halls, hospitals, law courts, police stations, fire stations and central government offices. And these local command centres are in continual communication with each other (sometimes slowly and sometimes more urgently). Each area of the 'city' has its own character and its specialist businesses, and yet each sector depends on every other sector. There is no real core intelligence at work, although some centres are more influential than others.

The key role of the limbic system

Perhaps the most influential structure in the body is the limbic system, which resides in the middle of your skull. The limbic system is a loose set of structures that are sometimes called the 'Emotional Brain', although it does a lot more than produce emotions.

Here is a list of the primary structures and I invite you to ask yourself, as you read through the list, what all these functions might have in common (clue: the answer is not 'emotion').

Thalamus. Processes information from the senses (notably sights and sounds) and turns it into crude data.

Hippocampus. Compares the data from the Thalamus to its library of cellular memories for matches to other significant experiences, and sends on its conclusions to the hypothalamus, the amygdala and the frontal lobes.

Cingulate gyrus. Allocates emotional responses to incoming data, and to autobiographical memories.

Amygdala. These twin structures are integral in releasing emotion through the nervous system. Also creates short-term shock/alarm reactions in an emergency.

Limbic system

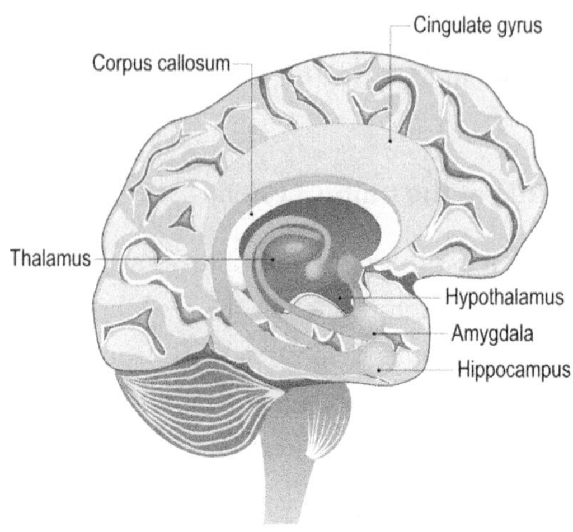

Hypothalamus. The size of a small nut, it orchestrates the action of every gland in the body and can therefore influence every organ in the body. Sometimes called the 'Master Controller'. Releases emotion but also controls temperature, sleep, water retention, endorphin release and the body-clock. Plus hunger, thirst, mood and the sex drive.

Did you identify anything in common between all these functions?

To my mind, what they have in common is that they all have something to do with adapting the body to the environment. Suppose, for example, you are a soldier manoeuvring through the desert. The limbic system will open the skin pores and sweat glands to regulate your temperature and increase water retention. Expand your power of attention to changes in the environment. Release fear to tell you to be watchful for the enemy. Scan minor changes in the environment for signs of threat. Shock you to get out of the way when that scorpion scuttles underneath you.

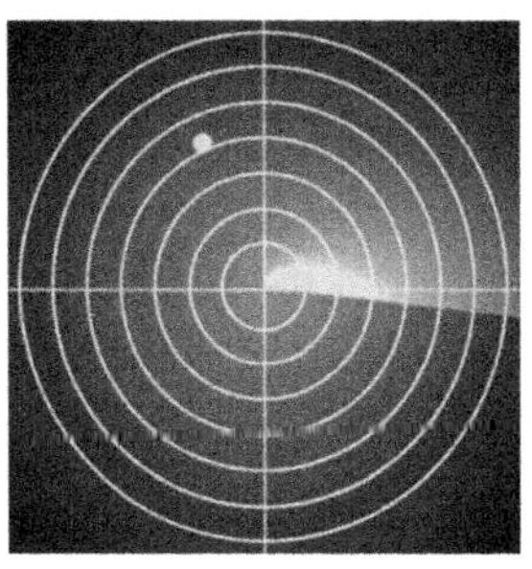

One metaphor for the limbic system is that it works like a radar station which monitors both the external environment and the internal environment (your thoughts, feelings, moods, heart rate, gut reactions, etc). It also examines how well your internal reactions are helping you to adapt to the environment you are in. Clearly your reactions to fighting in the desert would not be appropriate if you are having a picnic with your family, and vice versa. Think, also, of this internal radar as having radio access, telephones, email servers, and even couriers so that it can send out information to other areas in the 'city' and to your thinking centres. If the thinking mind works particularly well, it might even come up with some fresh strategies that help the body adapt better, or which will change the external environment.

Emotional production is an important task carried through by the limbic system, yet it is easy to see how that fits with the general purpose of the radar station. Emotions are your body's 'opinions' about what is going on out there: sad, funny, dangerous, relaxing, loathsome, shocking or plain crazy. So emotions are there to tell you what kind of experience you are having so that you can adapt all the better to it.

For example, someone shouts at you. Before you are conscious of the fact, the thalamus has already registered that there is a red face moving towards you, the noise is loud, and your personal space is being invaded. Immediately the amygdala presses the alarm button on the Sympathetic Nervous System and arouses you for action. Meanwhile, the hippocampus matches information from the thalamus against experiences of teachers/parents shouting at you, and signals the cingulate cortex to prepare a fear response (or an anger response, or both). The hypothalamus pulls together all these responses and triggers wholesale changes to the nerves, gut, muscles, skin and circulation which support the proposed reactions. At this point it is vital that the thinking mind is wide awake and attuning to these changes in the body, and quick off the mark with decisions: taking evasive action, self-assertion, speaking up, calming people down, etc. Or further distress will be sure to follow.

Bodymind and the emotions

Bodymind uses emotions in order to ensure both short-term and long-term survival. In the short-term it sends emotions like anger, fear and disgust in order to guide, warn and protect. In the long-term bodymind promotes emotions like joy (linked to endorphin release) whenever it notices that we are pursuing activities that improve health, raise self-esteem or are self-actualising. As I mentioned before, healthy people are happy people. When happy, such people do things for themselves and others that provide further emotional rewards.

Let us look at the different emotions Bodymind uses to promote short-term survival:

Fear. Bodymind wants us to reduce vulnerability, either for ourselves or for others. This might involve getting help, finding out the facts about the situation, reducing challenges down to smaller steps, and then taking those steps one by one until the problem is faced down - or escaped quickly, if we are talking about danger from knives, guns and bombs.

Anger. Bodymind wants us to assert our rights against a person or a group who are acting disrespectfully. This can involve speaking up constructively, organising opposition, or getting together with others who share our concerns. Bodymind does not wish us to blow up in rage (for that makes the situation worse, not better) but to be calm, specific and clear about what we want to see happening.

Sadness. Bodymind is alerting us to the fact that we have lost, or are about to lose, something, or someone, of deep importance to us. It is prompting us to fill the gap created by drawing closer to other people and getting comfort from them, before moving on to find a new equilibrium. Bodymind does not want us to go through a 'grief' process in which we get stuck in the past, for that does nothing to help us move on. The 'grief process' is largely an invention of psychologists who have failed to understand the nature and purpose of sadness, or emotions in general.

Disgust. Bodymind wishes us to distance ourselves from a threat – or better still, withdraw from it altogether. This could be poisonous food and animals, or it could refer to toxic people.

Frustration. This feeling state does not appear in some standard lists of emotions. I believe it to be a common emotion with an important message. It is also the only emotion which is pointing at you as well as at other people. The message of this emotion is to disengage from situations which you cannot influence and over which you have no control – including those situations you think you have to control. This may relate to unreasonable people, in which case your body is telling you to move away from a potential shouting match and reconsider that relationship. It may also relate to unreasonable demands that **you** are making on the people around you. We see this in control-freaks who sound their horns at other drivers in their way, fume at delays, and throw tantrums when they don't get their own way. In that case your body is asking you to disengage from the self-judgments in your head, on which, more later.

Excitement/Joy. Bodymind is confirming that we are doing things (or engaging in relationships) that are absolutely right for us. It is also urging us to share our pleasure and satisfaction with other people, thereby deepening our relationship with them. This sharing response can work in reverse as we take joy in the happiness of friends, family and community. Either way, sharing reinforces the emotion. The regular production of excitement and joy are vital to health because they confirm we are on the right road to self-actualisation and, as we saw earlier, self-actualising people are healthier people.

It is important to realise that there is no such thing as a 'negative' emotion. All emotions are positive in that they have a purpose: either to protect us or else encourage us to pursue the good life. Some 'emotions' considered negative are not really emotions at all, but products of 'Junk-mind': anxiety, grief and rage being just three examples. Others are thought to be negative because we are conditioned to believe that expressing them is 'weakness'; which is why so many of us bottle up fear and sadness. Conversely, other types of conditioning forbid the expression of anger, as doing so is considered bad manners.

Here is a list of pseudo-emotions alongside the genuine emotions with which they confused:

Anxiety - confused with Fear where anxiety comes about from worry and wrong work of the mind.

Rage - confused with Anger, where an outburst of rage is what (eventually) happens when you don't deal with your emotions.

Addiction - confused with Joy. Addictions occur when the person cannot let go of something which gives him pleasure, and keeps on demanding another 'fix'.

Grief - confused with Sadness, where grief refers to the inability to let go.

Genuine emotions such as fear, anger and sadness have a natural action cycle starting when bodymind first registers that we face a challenge, to completion of the actions it wants us to take in order to restore equilibrium. This is illustrated in the four steps that follow:

- A situation of concern is evaluated by bodymind (e.g. abusive people)
- An emotion is created in order to prompt for action (e.g. anger)
- Person takes appropriate action (e.g. speaking up)
- At this point bodymind checks that situational needs (e.g. your rights reinstated) are satisfied, and closes out the emotion.

OR

If we take no action (or words remain unvoiced) then bodymind 'turns up the volume' on the emotion and the emotion remains in force, typically getting stronger as time goes on.

Note here that emotions are not closed out until action is taken. As I shall explain later, unresolved emotions create a build-up of tension which results in bodily distress, and the potential onset of illness.

How does bodymind monitor situations and create the associated emotion? There are several mechanisms for this:

1. *Processes sensory information.* This is performed by the thalamus. Coded information about sights, sounds and other sensations are forwarded to the hippocampus, the hypothalamus and also to the thinking centres for further evaluation.

2. *Matches information about emotional experiences from the past using cellular memories.* Inside the limbic system are the cingulate gyrus and the hippocampus. These sites store information about all past significant emotional experiences. As situations arise, the hippocampus checks the incoming sensory information and matches it to a cellular memory of similar experiences (if it has one). It then triggers an emotional release based on the cellular memory.

3. *Super-fast activation of the glands and other message centres.* Bodymind uses the hypothalamus along with the amygdala to create and shape emotions. It creates a cascade of feelings, partly through the vagus nerve which runs along the spine, and partly through the action of the HPA Axis in which the adrenal glands change the activity of the autonomic nervous system. With multiple impacts on the heart, circulation, gut, skin and muscles. However, the hypothalamus can also influence the release of dopamine, serotonin, and GABA, which are messengers that influence emotions and mood.

Candace Pert, in her influential book *Molecules of Emotion* describes how the body uses peptides to create and store emotional codes in cells distributed throughout the body. 'muscle memories' are created similarly.

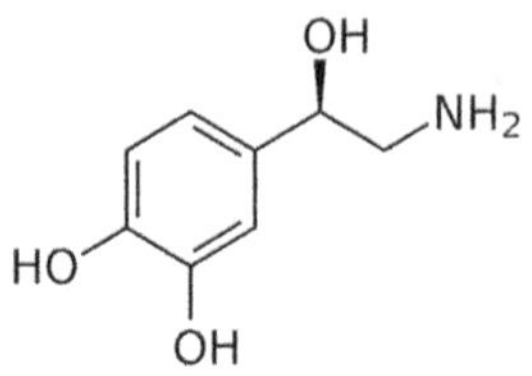

A peptide chain which stores information in the cells

Peptides are small protein chains that act as emotional messengers. These peptides bind on to cells in the brain and, interestingly, over 95% of them are found in the hippocampus. Peptides travel all over the body but are especially strong in the vagus nerve, the gut (the Enteric Nervous System), the skin, the muscles, and in all the major glands. Not only does the emotional brain 'tell' the glands, muscles and stomach what to do but they feed-back to it, and let it know how they are responding to that 'feeling'. This information is then used by the emotional Brain to either shut down the response, intensify it, or fine-tune it to optimise equilibrium. Candace Pert writes:

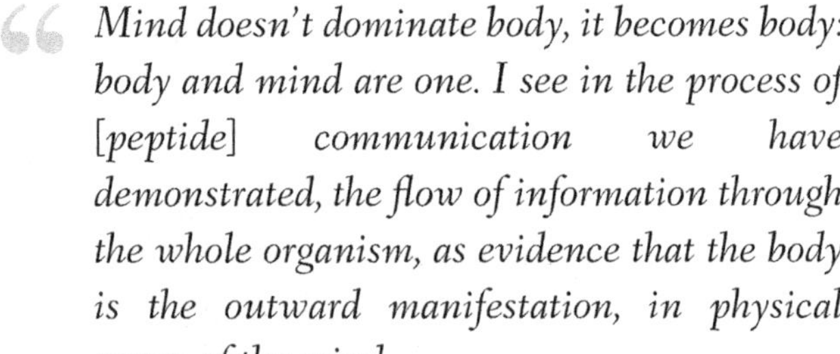

> *Mind doesn't dominate body, it becomes body: body and mind are one. I see in the process of [peptide] communication we have demonstrated, the flow of information through the whole organism, as evidence that the body is the outward manifestation, in physical space, of the mind.*

Emotional experience is complex and unique to the individual; in that way we learn to distinguish between different emotions and to sense the profound messages sometimes conveyed in them. While one person may register sadness via a rippling sigh and a loosening of the chest, another may recognise this same emotion, in a different key, via a blockage in the throat, a weight pressing down on the shoulders and oncoming tears. Not only do we differ from each other in our experience of emotion, but we may experience the same emotion in different ways, or in a cocktail mixed with other emotions.

Bodymind communicates to us every day of our lives. It acts like a guardian angel, alerting us to when we have a problem, sending an emotional signal and encouraging us to act in a way that preserves our own interests and the interests of those close to us.

Let us take some more examples from everyday life:

Anger. A friend calls and accuses you (wrongly) of criticising her behind her back. You try to explain, but she repeatedly interrupts you, her voice getting louder and louder. You experience an opening of the lungs, a rising feeling of force coming up through the chest, and tension in the jaw. Your body is encouraging you not to put up with any more abuse and tell your friend that she must either speak to you respectfully, or you will put the phone down.

Joy. You finally receive that long-awaited (and deserved) promotion. Your muscles relax, you feel lighter, and a warm feeling settles in your stomach. Your body is reinforcing your achievements and encouraging you to share them with people who care about you.

Fear. Tests reveal you need major surgery. You have never been seriously ill before. Now you are in unknown territory. Your body responds with increased heart-rate, stomach contractions, you swallow a lot, and your visual field closes in on you. Your body wants you to focus on what is about to happen to you, and take steps to adapt to this emergency, thus ensuring that you will receive the right care, and as much support as you can get.

Sadness. That dead-end relationship you have been in a for a few years finally breaks up and your partner moves out of the apartment. Although you feel relief, you also feel close to tears, for you are faced with living alone again. At least that relationship, while you were in it, gave you some intimacy. Your body now wants you to move closer to your friends and family for comfort and to find a way (eventually) to fill the gap.

Surprise. You are walking down the street and someone taps you on the back. You experience a mild shock running down your spine, you jump slightly, and your mouth opens. Your body is getting you to slow down, be careful, check out the situation and establish who it is that is communicating with you, and what it is they want.

Boredom. You have spent all day by yourself working on the computer, watching daytime television, or trawling the internet. You feel restless, 'flat' and yawn a lot. Your body is alerting you to the fact that you are low on stimulation, and need a change of scenery.

Disgust. You learn that someone you trusted has lied to you and stolen money from your bank account. Your nose wrinkles, your hands feel sweaty and you feel sick. Your body is urging you sever your connection to this person, and take steps to protect yourself.

As Antonio Damasio, the author of several important books on emotion, such as *Descartes' Error* has said:

> *Rather than being a luxury, emotions are a highly intelligent way of driving the organism towards certain outcomes.*

Notice that emotions always deal with situations that occur either in the present moment, or which are just about to happen. Emotions do not direct you to dwell on the distant past as, once the moment for action has passed, the emotional brain is no longer concerned with the issue. Bodymind does not actually 'think' in time: it only works in present moment awareness. You, the reader, may think that emotions can be about the past, but that is a misunderstanding. If you recall something that happened in the past and experience the emotions linked to that event, your body is really using its store of cellular memories to remind you of your emotional needs then, so that you can be better prepared to satisfy them now. For example, if you remember a car crash twenty years before and the fear you underwent, bodymind is actually using the emotional cue to remind you to be careful the next time you drive your car.

As a rule, people who dwell on painful memories are usually people who have not yet learned to forgive: resentment and bitterness are the usual result.

The case of Elliot

A real-life case cited by Antonio Damasio demonstrates what happens if we cannot connect to Bodymind and to our feelings, desires and emotions.

An operation to remove a tumour from Elliot's brain resulted in a loss of healthy tissue, which meant the connection between the frontal lobes (thinking centres) and the limbic system (emotional brain) was severed. The result was that Elliot could not access his emotions and intuitions. If shown gory photographs of crash victims, Elliot felt bored. Nor could he show much interest in images of beautiful, or touching, scenes.

Lacking access to his feelings, Elliot could not make decisions the rest of us would take for granted – like whether it was time to get up in the morning and meet a friend. In fact, he had not the slightest felt interest in events, whether good or bad. He saw no particular reason why he should do a job well (although he could understand – in theory – why it should be done). Nor did he have the emotional staying power to see a job through to the end. He made several poor decisions – based on his inability to 'read' his own and other people's motives – which led eventually to personal and business failure. Without bodymind to help him develop a feel for the right thing to do, he was helpless.

If the thinking mind denies access to emotion, not through an injury to the brain but through conditioning (e.g. 'don't make a fuss'), then those emotions have no place to go but back into the body, where they may fester for months, or years. Meanwhile, we might experience a seething, inner resentment, continually replaying the original scenario repeatedly.

William Blake's poem *A Poison Tree* springs to mind here:

> *I was angry with my friend: I told my wrath, my wrath did end.*
>
> *I was angry with my foe: I told it not, my wrath did grow.*

Blake describes how rage continues to fester, 'watered in tears' and 'sunned' with false smiles until it turned into a poisonous apple. At last the foe ate it and was found dead beside the tree. But it is unlikely that the narrator was emotionally healthier for that. If anger has gone on for too long then, if we have not taken the opportunity to speak up and resolve the matter when we had the chance, it is better to forgive.

In a later chapter I shall describe how emotions, when denied, can lead to the formation of symptoms in medically unexplained illness. Anticipating that argument, let us look at one case in which repressed emotions led directly to Fibromyalgia Syndrome.

Ann's case

Ann came to see me after suffering from Fibromyalgia for eight years. Reporting with muscle and joint pain over her arms, shoulders, back and upper legs. Additionally, with fatigue, headaches, vertigo and disturbed sleep.

We started by taking a careful case history, focusing on life-events that were occurring just before symptoms first appeared.

In Ann's case, there were three significant events. One was her mother's death, the second was a conflict with her sister, and the third was harassment from her in-laws. Initial (low-level) symptoms of pain occurred shortly after her mother's funeral.

The death of her mother deeply upset Ann. She lost her most important source of support, and her best friend. She did not think she would ever get over her death, or find anyone who could replace her; someone with whom she could talk on a deeper level about her feelings and concerns,

She was shocked and upset when her sister took away, without permission, all her mother's jewellery and tried to take possession of her house. From respect for her mother, and because she was scared of her sister, she said nothing. Her sister did in fact take the house, and Ann was still angry about this eleven years later.

Her husband's parents had always treated her poorly. Either ignoring her, or telling her what to do. Or else complaining to her husband about her 'attitude' until she learned to keep her mouth shut. In fact, they behaved in the same intimidating way as her sister. But without support from her husband (who told her he just wanted 'a quiet life') or from her dead mother, she felt unable to cope.

Ann knew vaguely that these factors had something to do with her illness but had yet to connect to her symptom message.

We worked together on making sense of this until we felt ready to put the message into words.

She then focused on her symptoms of pain and read out the following message:

'*My symptoms are here to tell me to stop hiding my emotions and start speaking up about them, politely, now!*'

On reading this, she became upset and talked about how much she loved and missed her mother. When this conversation concluded, we focused on preparing her for situations that required her to express her emotions.

On the third session, Ann reported her symptoms had been going up and down 'like a Yo-Yo'. Her journal showed, predictably, that symptoms had gone up when she took a phone call from her sister, when her in-laws dropped in one Sunday afternoon, and when her husband one night informed her, without discussion, that he had 'decided' that they would go on holiday to Cornwall that year.

Her pain went down again when she told her husband that if he wanted to go to Cornwall that was his choice, but she would not be going. If he wanted to go on holiday with her, she wanted to discuss other destinations so they could make the choice jointly.

They stayed down when she excused herself from her in-laws' company one Sunday, and took the dog for a walk.

Her relations with her elder sister took a while to resolve as she had always lived in fear of her, but she gradually learned to be more assertive and also wrote her a letter expressing her disappointment with her behaviour after mother's death.

She also realised her need for more emotional support. Prior to Reverse Therapy, she had been afraid of going out for fear of 'making the symptoms worse' but with returning confidence and improved emotional self-assertion, she spent more and more time going out with her friends (by the end of treatment she was about to embark on a ten day holiday with two of them to Minorca). After a few months she was completely well.

Key points in this Chapter

- Bodymind 'thinks' through cellular communication between the brain, the nervous system, endocrine system, the heart, gut, muscles and immune system

- The limbic system can be compared to a 'radar station' that monitors the external and internal environment
- Bodymind continually seeks adaptation to evolving problems with people and situations
- Bodymind uses emotions to give us its felt 'opinions' about what is happening to us, and cues us for action
- Emotions are crucial to decision making, and we ignore them at our peril
- Unresolved emotions can, if left unresolved for too long, result in early warning symptoms

4

ABOUT THE CONSCIOUS MIND

Conditioning and the mind

The first thing to realise about the conscious mind is that it is stuffed full with things that we never put there. For example, you are currently reading this book in English. Yet the rules of grammar and syntax were acquired by the language acquisition device in your brain that was activated a few months after birth. When it switched on, it replicated the sounds and phrases made by the adults out there, and gradually pieced together the rules of language under which they were operating. So that by about the age of six, most of you could understand a basic form of the English language. This learning process was entirely automatic; outside conscious effort and control.

In the same way you also acquired the cultural and social patterns of these models, along with many of their rules, judgments, beliefs, assumptions and expectations. You continued to accumulate these as you went through school, college, university, work and beyond. For some people this ends in conformism, even slavery. For others, it might be a stepping stone to something more liberating.

I described earlier the function of cellular memories in bodymind as cues for emotional responses. The equivalents in the thinking mind are cues for judgment. Many judgments based on memory and conditioning are practically useful. For example:

- Deciding what move to make next in a game of chess
- Knowing how to write an email
- Negotiating your way around the transport network
- Interpreting facial expressions
- Following a dress code
- Guiding your children towards good behaviour

However, for every useful judgment stored by the mind, there will be at least two that are less than useful, if not downright harmful. It is these I want to draw your attention to later in this chapter. Distinguishing between the two plays an important part in your emotional health.

To a great extent the mind is not personal; it does not truly belong to us. In some respects we can compare it to an internal judge, put there at an early age to ensure that we grew up knowing the rules. But in other respects it is like a library stocked with books, CDs and DVDs compiled by someone else. Although we are free to obey or disobey the rules, and free to use, or not to use, the records placed at our disposal, we are not free to create the records themselves. At least not until we get to adulthood, when it becomes possible to add to the store, and to change some (but not all) of them.

Let us look at some examples of this conditioning process.

Ethics. Assuming that the family and community you grew up in were law-abiding and conscientious, you will have grown up with a store of moral instructions that guided your behaviour. Some of these rules, such as 'do not kill' are advantageous to all, others ('my country right or wrong') are debatable, while others are merely arbitrary ('always do what your elders tell you'). With maturity, we can examine some of these moral rules and decide how far we are going to follow them. But we cannot escape them altogether.

Rituals. Children spend a large part of their early years watching what other people do. In this way they acquire a stock of procedures which help them become just like everybody else. Eating with a knife and fork, dressing up, writing with a pen, riding a bike, etc. Some rituals we observe and copy may be less benign: smoking, drinking, bullying, and our parents' Saturday night arguments.

Beliefs. It is strange to think that many thoughts we take for granted are not ours at all. After all, they are inside our heads, therefore do they not belong to us? Yet what many of them really are, are memes. Passed along the chain from one generation, one community, one family, to the next. Ending up in our heads. Like moral rules and rituals, some are useful, and some not. Later on in this chapter, we will look at some examples that are damaging to your health.

Imprints. These are episodic memories related to significant life experiences. Some of them shocking, some less so. All of them come with an emotional charge, so in some respects, they are shared by bodymind. However, where bodymind is primarily interested in the emotional lesson, the thinking mind relates them to the ego. An example of a positive imprint relates to when the child was held and loved. Negative ones relate to violence, abuse, rejection and anxiety, amongst other examples. Unfortunately, it is the negative ones that the ego remembers best. Recalling them, it builds negative beliefs based on them.

The ego is developed through several types of conditioning: parental, schooling, relationships, work and, finally, the negative judgments we gain unconsciously from the community in which we were raised. Let us look closer at these different sources.

Parental. Parents exercise influence over their children for better or worse, although this influence is not as profound as many people might assume. The fact is many of us outgrow our parents' influence, and many more still rebel against it. However, it is undeniable that parents (if they are not absent) contribute to conditioning. This may be benevolent: if the parents are admirable people the child may want to emulate them and will copy their excellent qualities, and that is what most of us mean by good parenting – that they are good models. But what about the poor ones?

Our parents (assuming that they actually take responsibility for our welfare) are, like us, only human, and they make mistakes. They are also subject to conditioning, irrational thinking, anxiety and delusions, just as we are. So your parents may have tried to be 'perfect' parents, and smothered you with their attention. Or they may have taken little interest in you because that was the way their parents treated them. They may have developed rigid ideas about how 'good' children should behave, and not made sufficient allowance for a child's waywardness; so you experienced them as hard, controlling and punitive. Growing up with a harsh ego and the guilt, perfectionism and worry that came with that. Or they may have thought children should be spoilt; so you grew up with the idea that the world should conform to your wishes – setting you up for the confusion, disappointment and frustration that came with that ego-position, when the world showed you otherwise.

Children instinctively and unconsciously (at least until puberty) model their parents' thoughts, communications and behaviour, and accept them as if they were normal, no matter how freakish they in fact might be. Because this modelling process is so subtle and uncritical, children cannot get any distance from their parents' example, and their ability to appraise those models does not appear until they have become adults themselves. By which time our parents' judgments may have assumed the status of commandments rather than makeshift generalisations. To take one example from my experience: my parents, like most of their generation, thought it was embarrassing to discuss their emotions, and I grew up believing that emotions were things you did not speak about. This gave rise to many problems for me when I reached the teenage years, as I assumed that fear, anger and frustration, amongst other emotions, were things I ought to keep to myself. This led, in my case, to something like a near-breakdown at eighteen when I was going through the crisis I described in Chapter 1.

Fortunately, conditioning is reversible and we can learn to let go of absolute judgments and discover how to adapt more productively to the trials of life. It is easier to do this when we surround ourselves with partners and friends who can either teach us how to change through their own example, or encourage us to adopt new ways of thinking through affection and support.

Schooling. When I first practiced as a psychotherapist in the early 1990s I assumed, as many therapists do, that the primary source of poor experiences in early life comes from bad parenting, or from dysfunctional families. This, until recently, was due to Freud's influence. Freud and his followers believed that all psychological problems could ultimately be traced back to frustrated desires directed at the parents. My subsequent clinical experience has shown me that this is not in fact so and that the influence of schools, institutions and peer groups can be just as pernicious.

For example, bullying teachers and children are, to my mind, a prime source of distress in children and can lead to long-term confusion, self-doubt, anxiety and depression when they become teenagers, and to the negative self-judgments we are exploring here. More insidiously, some schools promote a narrow conformism which punishes or excludes children who are unusual in any way. Even where that is not so, children in schools often form tribes which attack children who do not speak, dress or think in the same way the artificial tribe does. The child is faced with the option of conforming to the tribe and adopting its narrow outlook, or being excluded and treated to the persecution of the rest. All this can lead to the fixed belief that the person is a freak, thus paving the way to difficulties in relating to others, and future anxiety.

Conditioning does not stop once we reach adulthood; it continues on until death, unless we learn the habits of reflection and critical thought, of independent judgment and the courage to be ourselves, freeing us from the power of the ego. The path to maturity is long, but easier to walk when we inspect and discard the negative judgments we carry around in our heads. It helps, too, if we cultivate our emotional intelligence.

Thus far I have attempted to show that what goes on in our minds is largely the creation of others, added to random experiences over the years. That, since we weren't responsible for our conditioning, we have no control over the rules, thoughts and memories stored in the mind. However, we can choose which thoughts and memories we want to pay attention to. We can also choose to critique the ideas and beliefs we have inherited. However, to do that we will also have to overcome the ego.

The ego and its demands

The ego is not, as many people think, '*Who you are*'. Rather, it is the person you think you ought to be. Originally, that was based on the person others thought you were, or what they wanted you to be. Our first primitive experience of this artificial self came about in childhood, when we encountered the gaze of parents, teachers, and other children.

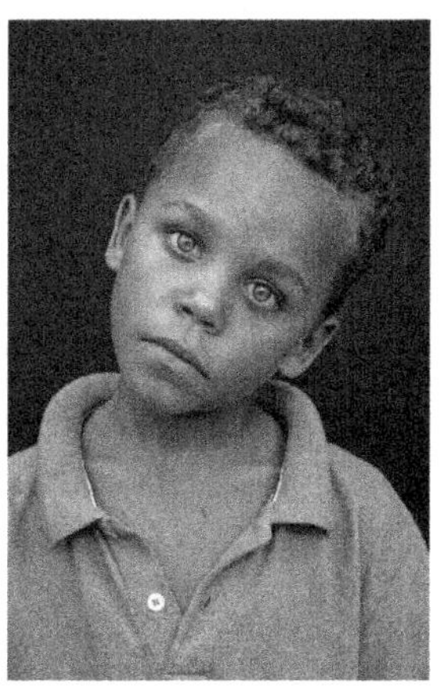

The Ego is first formed when the child meets the gaze of a parent and finds in it some idea of how he is perceived by others.

When we looked back into their eyes, we saw judgments of various kinds. If we were lucky enough to have attentive parents, then the first judgment we acquired was '*You are lovable*'. On that basis, the child's developing ego would have seen its first task as showing people how lovable it could be. Thereby receiving more love in return. Other judgments can help create a healthy ego if those judging us are kind, forgiving, and tolerant of the child's faults. By contrast, another child may encounter the judgment that she is unwanted. The ego created in that gaze, in that moment of shock, will withdraw from others. If the experience of rejection is continued, the child will grow up cold and unattached to people.

Unfortunately, the ego tends not to remember the good judgments well. It has better recall for the painful ones, which it sees as threats. Its way of dealing with these threats is to take over the negative judgment, and turn it back on the self as demands.

Here are some examples of punitive ego-judgments and their corresponding demands:

- You are not good enough - try harder
- You are weak - try to hide it
- You are stupid - you should just give up trying
- You are lazy - work harder!
- You are a nuisance - try to please people more

Notice that all these ego-demands are based on fixed beliefs about the self grounded on the judgments others made about us. Another way to think about the ego is that it is our internal judge. For some people, it can be merciless, and its constant demands, exhausting.

Built into the way the ego operates is magical thinking: the idea that thoughts control reality. One way this works is thinking that because we want something, we should have it. We can see this is in a child that throws tantrums when it does not get its own way. We see it also in the adult thrown out of a bar, drunk, for fighting the bar staff when refused more alcohol. However, there are more subtle examples.

A common problem that comes up with magical thinking relates to over-investment in outcomes. Say you are looking for a job. You scan the newspapers and the recruitment agencies for job opportunities, and find a position that's just right for you. Then you prepare meticulously. You look up the company's web-site, research its business operation, prepare for the first interview, put on your best outfit - and pass. You work even harder at the second interview, and make the short-list. At the third interview you make another good impression... but the next day you receive a phone call and learn you didn't get the job. Some people with small egos will accept this philosophically, moving on to the next search. But those with 'big', demanding egos may feel like it's the end of the world. The disappointment may be so great they give up searching. They may spend weeks chewing over what went 'wrong', or berating themselves for not doing more to get the position. They fell into the ego's trap of believing that because they wanted it bad enough, then it was sure to happen. In fact you were only ever responsible for giving it your best effort. The final outcome is not yours to decide.

Magical thinking is a distortion of consciousness. Because thoughts are in our head, the ego thinks they must be true, and that when we have them they must be pointing at something real. For example, your friend looks angry and up pops the thought that she is annoyed with *you*. Followed by a second thought that you must have done something wrong. If you take the trouble to ask her, instead of chewing over the 'insult', she tells you she is actually thinking about her ex-partner. As a general rule it is always a good idea to treat the thoughts in your mind with scepticism, until they are proven to have some basis in fact.

The feeling of anxiety that comes with some negative thoughts also reinforces the impression that the thoughts in our head must be true. After all, if we feel that bad about them then they must be true, right? In fact anxiety is an infallible sign that we are spending too much time in Junkmind. If a thought gives you anxiety then it is almost certainly an exaggeration of some kind, and a sign that you should be paying less attention to it, not more.

Ego demands, as thoughts often take the form 'I must...', 'I have to...', or 'I should'. Albert Ellis, a pioneer in cognitive therapy, conveniently called these thoughts 'musturbation'.

They are examples of distorted thinking, in which wishes have been escalated to final demands.

Examples include:

- I must get that job
- People must follow the rules
- I have to get it right
- I must not get angry
- They should know better

- I mustn't fail
- You should do as I say

Note, from the examples on this list, that these compulsions not only give rise to worry and anxiety, but also, when unsatisfied, create intense frustration. They can also poison our relationships with other people, when we apply musturbations to *them*.

The banana theory

In some parts of Africa and India, so far as I know, they still use an old-fashioned method to catch a monkey. The hunter will make a small wicker basket, with bars wide enough apart for a monkey's paw. Then he will find a grove where the monkeys live and put the cage on the ground, with a banana inside.

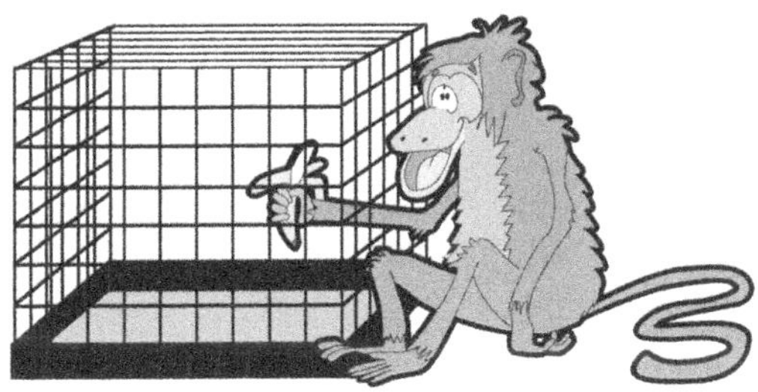

Then the hunter hides up a tree. Sooner or later some monkeys will come and inspect the cage. Finding the banana some (but not all) monkeys grasp it and hold on tight. But the bars aren't wide enough for it to withdraw its hand while still holding the banana. So it waits. And waits. It is still waiting when the hunter throws a net over it and hauls it off to the market.

We know a monkey's brain is only a little smaller than that of a human. You would think it was smart enough to let go of the banana. The reason it doesn't is not because it is stupid, but because its craving for the banana is stronger than its instinct for survival. The same principle applies to human beings. All of us have cravings - 'bananas' - we hold on to for dear life, even when holding on is against our best interests. One thing that stops people changing is worry about what will happen to them if they let go of the banana - they fear the loss of the Ego.

A banana is some rule or demand that junkmind tells us we have to have to hang on to, even when holding on to it brings us nothing but misery. It is a kind of fixation in which we imagine we have to try and live up to some impossible standard – 'lovable', 'successful', 'obedient', etc. These fixations are rooted in conditioning, and stored in the ego.

Here are some common bananas people have:

- I must be loved
- I have to be successful
- I should not show weakness
- I must have wealth
- I must be in control
- I should always know what to do
- I have to be admired
- I must not rock the boat

- I should not be sad
- I must not be selfish
- I have to do more for people
- I must not leave my comfort zone
- I should get well quickly

Note that these ego demands all involve 'musturbation'. It is ok to *wish* to be right, to be happy, to be loved and there is nothing in itself wrong with *wanting* to be a good parent, a caring partner, or a supportive friend. The problem arrives with the word must when we become obsessional about things and so the wish turns into a demand that something should always be the case. Before too long we are sacrificing every principle of sanity in pursuit of an impossible ideal.

Similarly there will always be times when life turns against us, we make mistakes, suffer financial loss or lose a partner. But if junkmind cannot accept that sometimes we are not good parents, that we won't have much money, or that we may have to be single for a while, then we are in trouble. We will brood instead of letting things go, rather like a junkie hurrying around trying to get his next fix. We end by overloading ourselves with burdens – giving in to our children's tantrums, working fourteen hours a day, or putting up with an abusive partner in order not to be alone. The more we try and hold on to the banana, the more we lose touch with ourselves and our deepest needs. Worst of all we end up feeling trapped, and the victim of circumstances when, in fact, it is the ego that has become our jailor.

In some cases, when we realise that our efforts earn us no thanks or gratitude, we might become resentful. Losing sight of the fact that no one ever asked us to hold on to that banana, we start to blame others for our suffering and, even, to get revenge through hurtful words and behaviour. Now we have added conflict with others to the list of stressors that we have to cope with.

How do we release a banana? The first step is to realise we have one. This can be difficult as we often see our own bananas as 'normal', as necessities that we and others could not live without. If they are pointed out to us, we may say things like 'But everybody wants more money!' or 'That's just the way I am – I can't say 'no' to people!' For many people their bananas are part of an unchangeable reality – just 'the way things are'. They miss the fact that, under the influence of other people's rules, and their own unconscious conditioning, they have become slaves.

One way out of the trap is to do the direct opposite of whatever we were doing while we were holding the banana. Instead of working more, we work less. Instead of seeking revenge, we ask for reconciliation. Instead of repressing our anger we find a way to express it constructively. Rather than pine for a lost relationship, we let it go. All these moves require that we take a risk and give up the ego – and the conditioning on which it is based. Many people find this difficult, and even scary at first. The reason for that is that they have confused the Ego with the Self.

Another reason for fear is that other people may have an investment in your banana, and it may upset them when you give it up. For example, if your banana is that you should always work hard, then it is a benefit to them if you do their work. Giving it up might mean that you forfeit their approval (many bananas are based on this). Nevertheless, that is a small price to pay if your aim is to get free of the ego, and become your own person.

Here is a personal example of this problem from my own history.

I grew up from the age of 3 with a partial hearing loss and spent years worrying about not being able to hear everything that was said (note the banana) and having to ask people to repeat themselves. To my mind being seen as deaf meant that I was also seen as 'stupid', as that was what I learned at school. This meant I had to work very hard to disguise my deafness and 'look intelligent'. I refused to wear my hearing aids in some places, which added to my problems.

After years of exhausting myself over this I decided one day – as a training assignment on a course I was taking - that I would go out without my hearing aids on a walk around central London. To my surprise I realised that, at least when shopping, very little hearing is actually required: you pick the items you want to buy, queue up, hand over your money, say 'thank you' and go. I even grew to enjoy telling people I could not hear well and asking them to speak up. I also realised that most people are very understanding when this happens and do not regard me as 'stupid' at all, so long as I explain about my hearing. After sufficient experience with people had taught me that 'deaf' does not always mean 'stupid', wearing the hearing aids became easier until nowadays, they mean no more than the shoes I am wearing. Years ago I could never have written about my handicap. The fact that I can do so in this book gives me, even now as I write, the good feeling that comes with self-acceptance rather than self-distrust.

The parable of the Two Zen Monks illustrates the power of these bananas perfectly.

Two Monks were on a pilgrimage to another monastery. They had both taken vows not to touch other people, and to remain silent at all times. After many days they came to a torrential river. On the bank was a beautiful young peasant girl who could not get across because the water was too deep. She asked the monks if one of them would carry her across.

The first Monk replied, 'All right', carried her on his back, set her down on the other bank, and wished her a safe journey. The two Monks continued on their route but the second Monk brooded. After they had walked on together for several miles he could no longer contain himself and burst out:

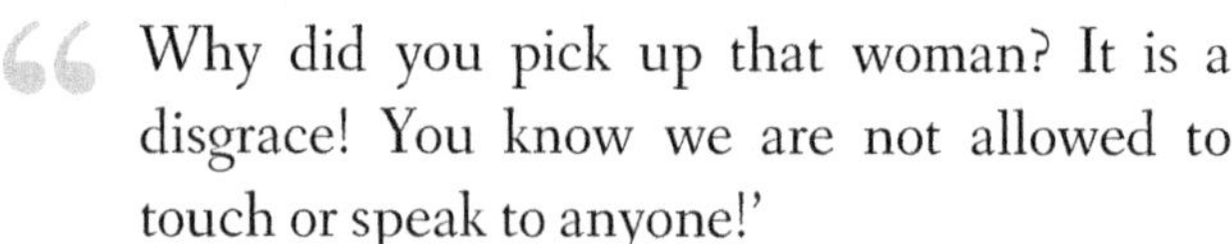

> Why did you pick up that woman? It is a disgrace! You know we are not allowed to touch or speak to anyone!'

Let it go, brother' said the first Monk, 'you're still carrying her.

Common ego patterns

No body of research has conclusively established that there is a fixed personality type which leads to disorders such as Chronic Fatigue and Fibromyalgia. However, in his book *When The Body Says No - Exploring the Stress-Disease Connection*, Dr Gabor Maté describes some interesting patterns. Dr Maté is a specialist in auto-immune diseases. However, his observations are equally relevant to the disorders we are investigating in this book.

Please bear in mind in what follows that all these patterns result from conditioning. Therefore they are reversible. However, I invite the reader to identify which of these patterns are based on ego-demands.

Weak boundaries. The individual has difficulty in distinguishing between her own needs and those of others. As a result, the individual becomes over-tolerant of people who take advantage. Often this pattern is formed in children with weak or demanding parents.

Low tolerance for uncertainty. The individual has an acute need for control and becomes anxious in situations where it is unclear what he should do next. Such individuals may also spend a lot of time worrying about the future. This comes up where too much is expected of the child.

Emotional suppression. Sometimes this pattern appears

as an inability to put emotions into words; or the words come out as thoughts rather than feelings. Other people have grown up without permission to speak about their emotions, so they sub-consciously tune them out.

People pleasing. This trait may be associated with blurred boundaries, leading to excessive compliance. People with this trait are 'too nice for their own good'. As children they were taught that doing what others want gets them attention and approval. Alternatively, it soothed adults away from criticising them.

Inability to say 'No'. This should be self-explanatory.

Perfectionism. The individual continually tries harder to get it right, to work harder, to be better. Her best is never good enough, and she is a workaholic. Linked to the belief that one must never make mistakes.

Over-conscientiousness. This is like perfectionism, except here the person is driven to prove themselves to others by taking on more and more demands, to the point of becoming overwhelmed. This especially relates to family, friends, and employers. Aside from anxiety, this is the only personality trait that is measured in personality tests.

Big Egos. Such people identify themselves as 'strong', proud people who do not need help from others and can bear any amount of responsibility (or distress). They also place a lot of demands on themselves. The result is they are over-burdened, isolated, and unable to ask for help when they really need it.

Poor adaptability. Due partly to their drive towards perfection and ego-strength, and partly because of their high need for control, these people find it difficult to adapt to adverse events. Since they also find it difficult to ask for help, they struggle on alone, until they are overwhelmed.

Anxiety. Surveys on individuals with Chronic Fatigue Syndrome, Fibromyalgia, IBS, Colitis, Auto-immune disease and similar conditions repeatedly show that patients score high on anxiety. Although sometimes anxiety is triggered by illness itself, many sufferers have a prior history of anxiety dating back to their teenage years. Anxiety is also measurable on personality tests, and there are several (free) ones available online.

More Females than Males. Surveys show that women outnumber men by a factor of 2 to 1 for most of the illnesses under consideration. Why this should be so is a mystery, as the triggers for these illnesses are more or less the same for everyone. Theories why this should be so include physiological differences, poorer conditioning for girls than boys, differences in gender roles, or because women are more likely to report these illnesses than men.

Broadly speaking, all these characteristics, except for gender differences, can be divided into three types: wrong ways of thinking, faulty relationship patterns, and Ego problems related to past conditioning. All of these are addressed in Reverse Therapy, as I describe below, in Chapter 6.

Differences between the right and the left brain

One thing to know about the brain is that the frontal lobes display two different types of thinking. To over-simplify for a moment, the right lobe (over your right eye-brow) is concerned with meaning, while the left lobe is concerned with facts. Confusingly, the right frontal lobe is governed by the left side of the brain and the left lobe by the right. Hence the (misleading) labels 'right brain types' (creative, intuitive, imaginative) and 'left-brain types' (factual, logical, analytical). While we need the right brain (left lobe) to tell us what things mean, or could mean, the left brain (right lobe) is telling us what is actually there. For example, the left brain processes that we are seeing a beach, and the sea, and a blue sky. Feeling the sun on our back, hearing the cry of the gulls and the laughter of people around us. The right brain notices that Bodymind is releasing excitement and joy, and computes that we are on the first day of our annual holiday, and it is time to party. So far, so good. When the two sides of the brain are collaborating well, and the right brain is staying close to the facts registered by the left brain, then not much can go wrong.

But let us look now at a sinister example in which the right brain is out of control

This time the left brain notices that we are entering a room full of people, most of them holding drinks and chatting. There are tables loaded with nice food and bottles of alcoholic drinks. Beautiful clothes and surroundings are all around. There is a hum of conversation and some laughter. Music is playing in the background and a few people are dancing. Some guests are smiling, others talking seriously. A few people turn to look at us as we enter the room...

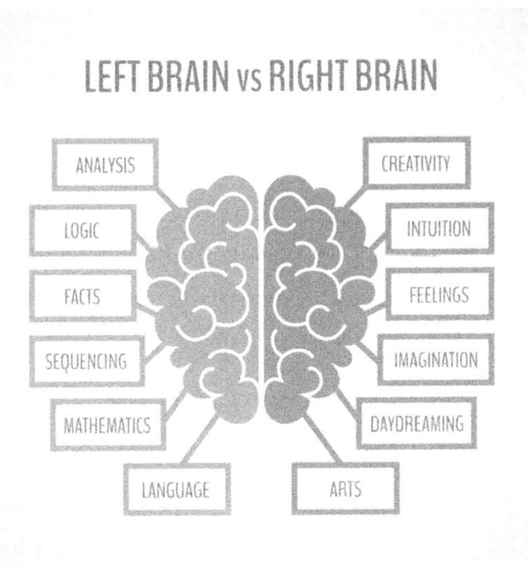

Although there is no such thing as 'left brain' and 'right brain' types, it is undeniable that there are significant differences in function between the two hemispheres.

This time the right brain thinks this is not a holiday occasion, but a nightmare. We won't know what to say, and people are hostile. Those people looking at us as we came in think we don't belong there. We came in the wrong clothes and look like freaks. We really should not be there at all. By now waves of anxious thoughts have reduced us to quivering wrecks, and we look for a quiet corner where people won't notice us. Shortly afterwards we have a panic attack, make our excuses, and go.

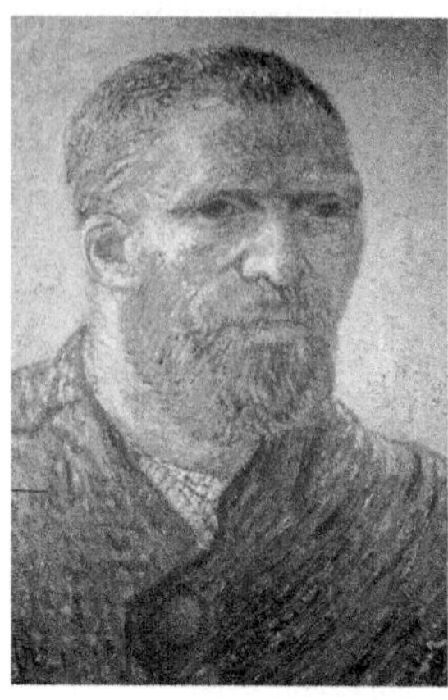

One of Vincent Van Gogh's paintings recently sold for $82 million. He also had numerous mental health problems: anxiety, depression, social isolation and alcoholism.

The right brain can turn heaven into hell. It is the seat of creativity, right enough and can be the source of originality, even genius. But equally so it can make us crazy, unless we stay grounded in what is actually happening, rather than what we imagine must be happening. Many imaginative, gifted writers and artists have also been crazy in actual life, to a greater or less degree.

This right/left brain split is widely misunderstood, giving rise to the myth that people are divided into 'left-brain' types and 'right-brain' types. In fact, nearly all human beings, whether male or female, use both sides interchangeably. It's just that some of us combine the two in the right way, and some do not. In decision-making, for example, both halves of the brain are important in coming to a best decision. We need the left brain to tell us the options before us, and the facts that support each choice, and the right brain to tell us what it might mean if we follow one option over another. And we need emotional cues feeding in from the limbic system to guide the choice.

Contrary to common belief it is the the so-called 'logical' left-brain, which has better connections to the limbic system and its emotional messages. It analyses feedback from the body relating to heart-rate, visceral reactions and nervous activity. That is because it is concerned with what is happening in the now, while the right brain focuses on what might happen next. Brain scans of people who are anxious, depressed or psychotic show that it is the right brain which is most activated. That is because distressed people are commonly pre-occupied with right-brain fantasies. By comparison, brain scans of people who are meditating show that the position is reversed: the left-brain is activated as you focus on the sights, sounds and feelings associated with the mindful state in the here-and-now. Although the right-lobe will eventually quieten down also, as those pesky judgmental voices die away.

Let us consider an example which could lead to bodily distress.

You are in the last year of your University Degree course, and several weeks behind on some of your assignments. You know you are weak in some subject areas, and you haven't yet decided what your dissertation is going to be about. The final exams are just three months away. You are confused and scared about the situation. Let us also assume that you haven't read this book, and are unaware of the action message supplied by your body, via the emotion of fear. Let us also assume that junkmind has hijacked your right brain. You then listen to that panicky inner voice passing on speculative judgments to you:

'You've run out of time now. It's too late to do anything about it'

'What a disaster! You tried to write that essay at two in the morning, but it's just not working'

'You'll never get a first now, and you absolutely must get a first'

'Your parents spent all this money on your education and you have let them down'

'Don't even think about asking for an extension. That would be weak, and then you really won't get a first'

'That tutor doesn't like you, so you can't go annoying her again'

'Anyway, you're cracking up. The stress is just too much'

'You might as well give up now'

'Oh well. It'll be a life-time flipping burgers'

Notice the panoply of worry, perfectionism, obsessions, guilt, bananas, and catastrophic predictions about the future. As well as blocked emotions and the refusal to ask for help. You can guess that this student will have acute anxiety and unresolved fear; two of the triggers for the illnesses we are explaining in this book.

Let us now consider how the same situation could pan out if this student's mind was working for her, instead of against her.

First, there would be no bananas about having to get top grades. There might be a wish for a first-class degree and a willingness to work hard for it, but it's a desire rather than a demand. There is also the accurate recognition that she will stand a better chance of achieving good grades if she stays focused.

The next step might be an acceptance of fear, the realisation that she can't do it on her own, and that help from other people is a necessity.

The next step might be a (left-brain) appraisal: How much work is there to complete? How much time is left to do it in? What are the first priorities? What are the options in getting help?

While this is going on the right brain will be coming up with some creative, 'out of the box' options for essays, dissertations, and short-cuts towards revision. In short, the right-brain will be focusing on possibilities rather than predictions of disaster.

Meanwhile the body will provide an 'opinion' about each of those options ranging from relief, and a push to explore the option in more depth, to a gut-feeling that the option simply won't work, and another option might be better. These emotional assessments will be accurately processed by both the right, and the left brain.

The following step might entail the formation of a plan, and the next step after that consultation with other people – lecturers, tutors and support staff – who can give professional advice. Meanwhile, our student is talking openly with her friends and family about her predicament and getting the nurturing and help that she needs during this tough time. At the same time, ensuring she is keeping the body working efficiently with regular hours, a healthy diet, exercise, and moments of quiet time away from work, as well as with her friends. If she is working with Reverse Therapy, I would ask her to practice mindfulness every day, in order to keep a distance from those panicky judgments.

Are you in your right mind?

Even the ego and its problems form only a small part of conscious activity. Mostly, the conscious mind is filled with random information taken from memories, books, television, the newspapers, the radio, the internet and from our interactions with other people. Making up a vast, ceaseless traffic of useless information passing through the mind every second, every minute, every day. And so we lose the ability to listen to ourselves.

There are around 86 billion cells in the brain and at least ten times that number of neural networks. The amount of information that can, potentially, pass through the conscious mind is practically limitless. One way to think about human beings is that we are fragile mammals with super-computers in our heads. And that computer is not under our control, either. The brain processes information and takes decisions outside our conscious control, later on presenting its decisions to the mind as a given, leaving us with the delusion that we made those decisions. Sometimes we are presented with two or more decisions to 'choose' from, but even in that circumstance we will typically select the decision the brain most wants us to take, employing emotions to guide us towards the decision it considers best suited to us.

Nor do we have much control over the thoughts themselves. From the moment we wake in the morning until twilight's last gleaming, a ceaseless flow of thoughts crosses in and out of consciousness.

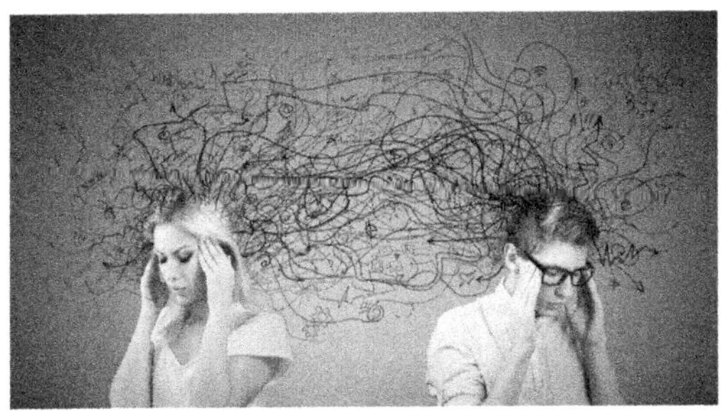

It has been estimated that the average person has around 10,000 thoughts a day. Without careful training 'Junkmind' can become quite chaotic.

Random thoughts followed by painful thoughts, hopeful thoughts, depressing thoughts. Then exciting thoughts followed by worrying thoughts, helpful thoughts, nonsensical thoughts. All of them bubbling up from somewhere deeper in the brain. Some are triggered by chance associations, some by memory, some by the task we are engaged in, some by conversation, while others come from the imagination. Few are of much practical use and most are from junkmind. Some of us will waste years ruminating over those same thoughts, despite the fact that most of them don't lead anywhere.

When the mind works properly, it works with conscious purpose and a focus on concrete aims. It is a marvellous tool through which we can speak and write, explain ourselves, exercise creativity (within bounds), interpret events, understand problems and formulate plans. It is also, when rightly directed, good at exercising emotional intelligence (i.e. noticing the emotional cues bodymind is using to guide us towards the right decision).

Unfortunately, some human beings are neither rational, nor emotionally intelligent, and are at the mercy of junk-mind. Realising how much it controls us may be the first step in gaining freedom from it - and getting our health and sanity back.

Junkmind is that part of the thinking mind which is filled with random information, irrational ideas and wrong conditioning. It is stuffed with negative thoughts: worries, obsessions, guilt, control-freakery, perfectionism, paranoia and other delusions. It can live in the past (wondering about all those 'what ifs') or hallucinate the future (usually in the form of disaster movies). Typically, it is a frightening place to be. And it is useless for working with bodymind because our emotional intelligence is just too subtle for it, and because junkmind sees emotions as a puzzling nuisance.

Worry - enemy No. 1

This chapter can only offer a limited purview of the many problems created in junkmind on which another, fairly large, book could be written. Here our focus remains on the problems which give rise to bodily distress. Of these, the greatest is worry.

A worry is a catastrophic judgment about you, your friends and family, or the problems which may befall you, or them. Typically, it is an exaggeration of some kind. For example:

'I am a failure'

'They hate me'

'Something terrible is going to happen now'

'I can't cope with this much longer'

'Nobody understands me'

'I'll never get over it if anything happens to her'

'I will never be well again'

We should distinguish worries from descriptions, which may or not be true. So you may have failed an exam, but that does not make you a failure. Your partner may have said hurtful things to you; that does not mean she doesn't love you. You may have been ill for four years; that does not mean you will never get well.

We should also distinguish worries from concerns. Worries are delusions you can do nothing about; concerns are matters which you can influence. You may be overwhelmed with responsibilities and in order to learn how to cope with them you may have to reduce them first. Your colleagues at work may not understand what you are asking for, and you may have to find another way to make them understand. You may be so ill you are in constant pain, and yet you can search for the right treatment for your Fibromyalgia. The difference is this: concerns are things you can actually do something about; worries paralyse your ability to act. One way to dispel a worry is to take action on the underlying concern. This gives the thinking mind a focus on solutions, rather than catastrophes.

If you are bothered by negative thoughts, then the long-term remedy is to practise ignoring them until they extinguish. The oxygen for alarmist thoughts is attention; the more time we spend wondering about them, the bigger they grow. Conversely, when we cease to pay attention to them, they wither away. You can demonstrate this fact for yourself by considering the worries you used to have as a child or a teenager, but which do not bother you any more. For example: that you would never learn to ride a bike because you kept falling off? Never get over having to wear teeth braces? That you would fail your exams?

Those are common examples, to which you can add to your own long-forgotten store of useless worries. But what they all have in common is that what seemed real to you then, now seems quaint.

There was a US survey many years ago which investigated the unreality of worries. In the survey thousands of adults were asked to describe the things they were worried about, and write them down (this is important because, very often, people forget what they were worried about a few days later). A few months later the respondents were followed up and asked how far their worries had come true. About 90% of them reported that the things they were worried about had not, in fact, happened at all. A further 7% were worries that had happened to some degree, but not nearly to the extent dreaded. This left only 3% of worries which had some basis in fact. As I often point out to my clients, if we focused our energies on managing that 3%, instead of wasting time on the others, we would easily overcome genuine problems.

It comes as a surprise to a great many people when they take the trouble to write down their worries, and compare those predictions to the final outcome a short while later. When I tried this myself many years ago I collected about a dozen paper slips and put them in my desk drawer. Weeks later I looked at those slips again and had a hard time remembering what many of them were about. You can try this for yourself.

Blocks to emotional expression

The ego – if so conditioned – may disconnect from emotions on the view that they are weird, irrational or intrusive. Typically this idea goes back to early-life experiences in which we modelled other people who were in emotional denial at the time. In extreme cases this can lead to a problem called *Alexithymia* in which we cannot actually recognise an emotion when it comes up in the body. We may experience it as indigestion, or as a heart palpitation for example. Or otherwise as a strange fluttering, breathless, agitated state which we cannot account for. And if we cannot *recognise* an emotion then we cannot give it a name, and we cannot know what to do about it.

More commonly, people *do* know when they are having an emotion, but react to it as if were something undesirable to have: plain bad, selfish, weak, or else childish. Junkmind has decided that expressing emotions will damage our relationships with other people when the exact truth is the opposite: correct and constructive channeling of the emotions will improve our relationships (or at least make them more realistic, and consequently more mature).

Fairly often, the ego denies emotion because it worries that we will be rejected if we follow our own emotional truth. This in turn arises from experiences in which we observed other people speaking up about their feelings, only to be met with scorn or dismissal. Another source of denial comes about from observing adults mis-handle anger, as when parents get into a rage with each other. Now, as we saw earlier, rage is what happens when emotions are denied, building up to such a point that we explode over relatively minor frustrations. Unfortunately the child mistakes rage for anger, and is so disturbed by it that she silently concludes that she must never get angry with anyone. On similar grounds fear, sadness and frustration may be denied because they attract negative judgments from other people who judge us as self-indulgent or 'neurotic'.

Specifically, junkmind interferes with emotional expression by:

- Assuming that emotions are unreal, and thoughts the only true reality
- Treating emotions as weird, or dangerous
- Applying rules which deny permission for emotions to be expressed
- Thinking we must be 'bad' if we focus on our own needs
- Blaming others for our 'negative' emotions ('if it wasn't for you...')
- Sitting on the emotions for so long that we become ill
- Worrying about what might happen if we do express emotion

Junkmind interrupts emotional expression in three ways: denial, rationalisation and anxiety. Let's look at examples of all three interruptions in action:

Denial. In this mechanism junkmind acts as if the emotion is not there, or else that it shouldn't *be* there. In the first case the individual may not actually notice the emotion, as he is consumed by traffic coming from the mind which over-rides potential awareness. We say of such people that they are 'stuck in their heads'; trapped in thoughts that distract them from the emotional truth. In other cases we may be partially aware of the emotion but that awareness is interrupted by injunctions like: 'whatever you do, don't go *there*!'

Example. We are stuck in a deadening life-style and we are provided with an opportunity to take a new job, or some other opportunity which fills us with excitement. The message from bodymind is for us to take this opportunity seriously. But junkmind disconnects from that emotion as to follow it would 'too risky', 'selfish', or would mean asking for help. If you are holding bananas that compel you to remain 'strong' and not ask others for help, then your excitement might appear very dangerous indeed. Nevertheless, unresolved emotions will remain in the body waiting to be understood and expressed, and for you to make your decision.

Rationalisation. In this mechanism junkmind comes up with specious reasons which explain away the reasons for having the emotion, with the implication that emotions are misguided, and should be ignored.

Example. A teenager is rude, nasty and selfish. Inwardly we feel angry and frustrated. But junkmind thinks we will be an bad parent if we call for some respect, and triggers a process in which we rationalise thus: 'she's having a hard time at school' or 'he's going through that difficult phase' or even 'they're good children really'. And so the child's bad behaviour continues, leading to still more frustrating encounters.

Anxiety. In this mechanism the experience of emotion is immediately replaced by the anxiety state, in turn triggered by alarming thoughts. Sometimes junkmind is alarmed by the fact that emotions exist at all in what should be a neat and tidy world. More often it thinks that *talking* about emotions honestly would be damaging to the Ego, and worries what people would think if they were expressed.

In some cases the anxiety response is automatic and the individual freezes when encountering threatening situations. This 'freeze' response is created by the Vagus Nerve when prompted by the Amygdala. Most often it is the result of bullying, or a traumatic incident in earlier life such that the person believed they were helpless to protect themselves at that time. That idea has become so engrained that the vagus nerve over-reacts to even mildly threatening incidents in the same over-the-top fashion.

Such long-term conditioning can be unlearnt in therapy, although it will take time to retrain the vagus nerve to tone down its reactions. This is the nerve that runs all the way down from the brain stem, along the spine, and then to your nervous system and enteric system. It is the key to the so-called 'fight/flight' response, although that term is an over-simplification, as the recent work of Stephen Porges has shown.

Interestingly, it has been recently discovered that it can be simpler to retrain the vagus nerve using breathing techniques, so that it ceases to unleash either the alarm response, or the freeze response.

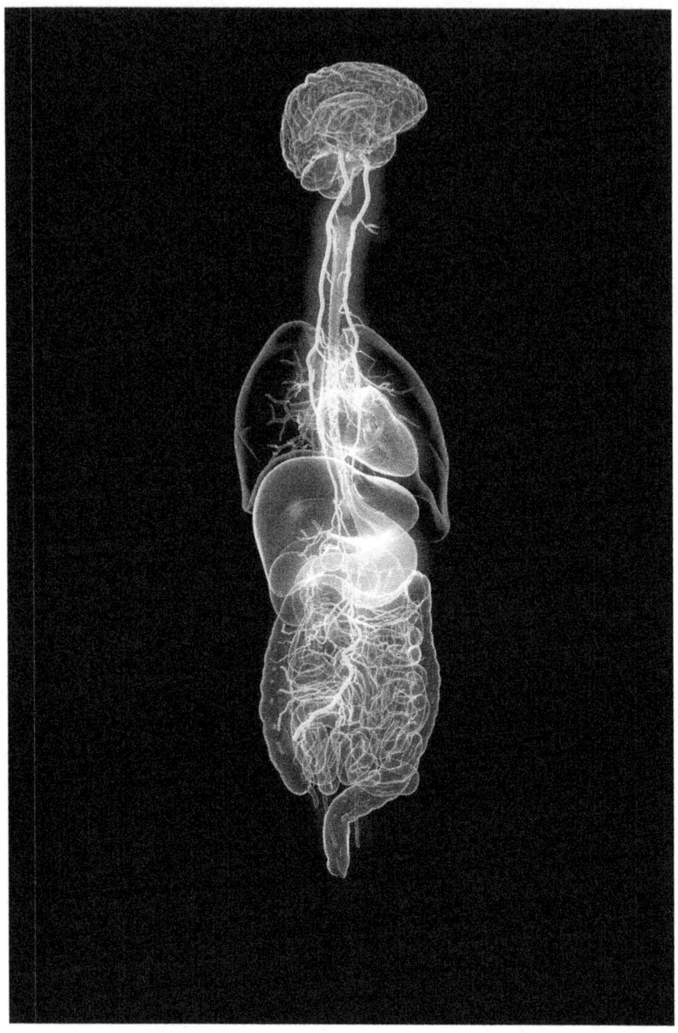

Stephen Porges' Polyvagal Theory has changed our understanding of how the Vagus Nerve works. Showing us that it is capable of three responses: the Alarm response (fight/flight), the Freeze response, and the Engagement response, in which we are cued to slow down, explore feelings, and talk things through.

Left entirely to its own devices junkmind could succeed in turning life into a hell of anxiety or else into a deadening, boring, routine, in which emotions are suppressed and nothing new or exciting ever happens. This is one reason why young children, who are much more attuned to the body than we are, become bored easily – their natural curiosity resists sameness. Emotions, for them, are pathways to new forms of action. If we adults listen to junkmind too often then we lose the balance between what is right for us personally, and what is right for others. At that point we become over-concerned with doing things right, instead of doing the right thing. A good example of this relates to people who become ill in stressful jobs. Stuck in the tunnel-vision of junkmind they become pre-occupied with security, making money and getting ahead. Since they have little time left over for relationships or leisure time their families suffer as much as they do. Life has become Work and its emotional point has been lost.

Making the mind work for you

Do you control your mind or does your mind control you? Or are you in control most of the time, but sometimes find that you get hijacked? This section describes how you can stay in control. For the mind is a good servant but a terrible master.

Referring back to earlier sections in this chapter, here are some signs that indicate that you have lost control:

- You are stuck in automatic reactions you inherited from others
- Driven by ego judgments, demands, and bananas
- Spending too much time over-thinking memories and thoughts that lead nowhere
- Plagued by worry and anxiety
- Guilt, self-blame and other negative self judgments
- Burdened by perfectionism, people-pleasing and other unhealthy patterns
- Difficulty in relating to your emotions
- Disconnection from the body and numbness, boredom or emptiness
- 'Always crashing in the same car' - making the same mistakes over and over again

The first step to taking control is to change your relationship to the mind. Seeing it as a tool for use by you when needed, to be put back in a box when not. Use it the same way you would a computer: switching it on when you want to write something, send and receive messages, or extract information. Then switching it off when the task is completed.

The second step is be sceptical of your thoughts. Working on the assumption that the majority of them are trivial, useless, or downright harmful. Understanding that thoughts are not facts; they are just thoughts. That the mind is not an infallible guide to reality, but, at best an interpreter - and a wayward one at that. Be constantly mindful that much of what goes on in the mind is either wrong, biased or delusional and that, most of the time, you should pay little attention to it. In short, you must become a thorough-going sceptic like the philosopher, Montaigne, who wrote:

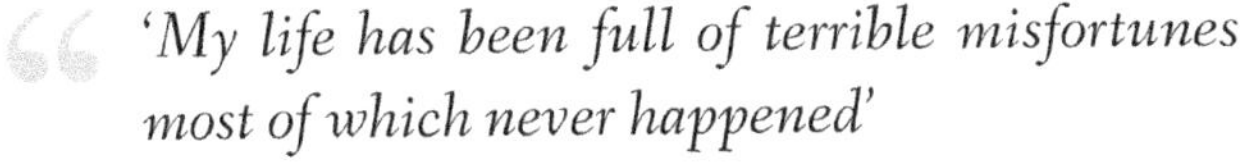

> *'My life has been full of terrible misfortunes most of which never happened'*

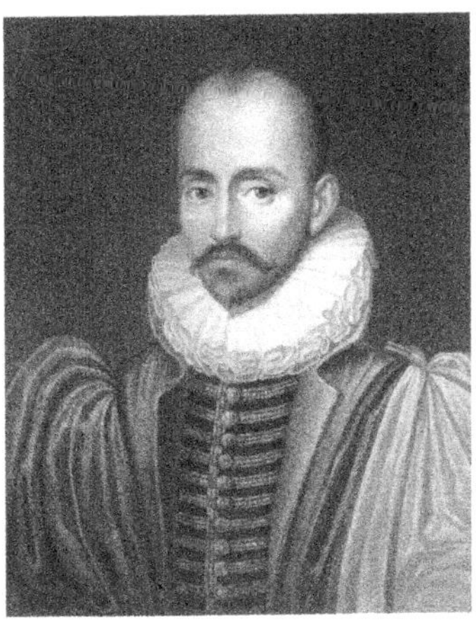

Michel de Montaigne (1533-1592) argued that our thoughts are an unreliable guide to reality and should be treated with caution. The motto on his coat of arms read 'Que Scais-Je?' (What do I really know?)

Montaigne tells us that people frequently get lost in words and in theories, when they would be better off examining the facts and noticing what is happening around them. He also suggested that people should get out of their heads and learn to live in present moment awareness - something we are rather keen on in Reverse Therapy.

The third step is to be selective about the thoughts you pay attention to. The secret to making your mind work for you is to live in the moment as much as you can, attending to your concerns, wishes and emotions day-by-day on an adaptable, problem-solving basis, while staying out of junkmind as much as possible.

Here are some rules you can follow which show when you should be in thinking mind, and when not. If any of the following apply then you can go ahead. If not then you should disengage from the thinking centres and focus your attention elsewhere.

- Do you have a specific problem that requires a solution?
- Do you have a concern which relates to matters you can actually do something about?
- Do you want to work on a specific goal so that it is measurable, actionable and realistic within a time frame?
- Do you have a decision to make?
- Do you want to make plans?
- Do you want to establish how something works, or why it is happening?
- Are you engaged in fact-finding research?
- Are you engaged in a creative project?
- Do you need to prepare a spoken or written communication?

The golden rule is that thoughts should have a goal or a purpose. If neither is present, you are most likely in junkmind.

When the thinking centres are working properly (meaning that the mind is now your servant), you have access to a powerful store of practical knowledge based on experience and observation. You also have access to a super-computer designed to process information and generate conclusions at amazing speed. The mind is also a critical tool for use in examining faulty ideas and judgments, and replacing those with better ones.

In relation to the main subject of this book, thinking mind, when under your control, is a necessary aid to maintaining health and sanity. In the final chapter I refer to the subject of resilience, which is the art of managing difficult life events. Anticipating that discussion, I list here some of the ways in which the mind, with its practical, problem-solving intelligence, exercises resilience:

- Distinguishing between problems we can solve, and those we can't
- Keeping a sense of perspective (for all life-problems will fade, eventually)
- Establishing the facts
- Selecting realistic goals
- Setting limits to what we can do
- Making decisions and formulating plans
- Finding new solutions to old problems
- Seeking help
- Adapting, as people and situations change

- Communicating clearly
- Putting emotions into words
- Paying attention to bodymind

Paying attention to bodymind

Suppose you are taking a walk in the woods and notice a strange coloured 'rope' in the grass. Let us suppose for a moment that you are not connected to your emotional brain, and you have to rely solely on thinking mind to help you work things out. Because the conscious mind works relatively slowly compared to bodymind, you stare at the thing for some time and notice that it has some strange, zig-zag marks on it, and also it has a green-brown colouring.

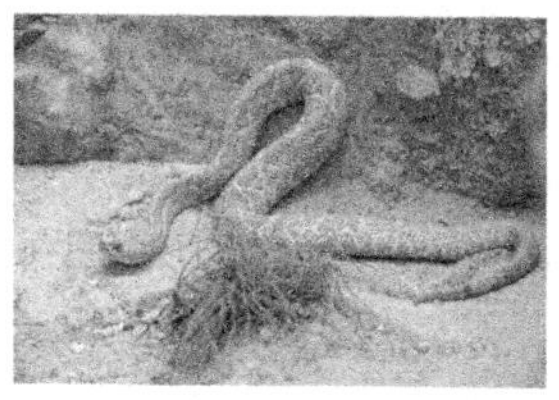

A snake can move faster than the eye can track, but not faster than the emotional brain can detect it.

You wonder whether some children have been painting coils in the forest, or whether someone has lost an ornament. You might theorise about ancient, pagan cultures that created the totem as part of their tribal rituals, and wonder whether you have made a unique discovery. Suddenly, the 'rope' moves towards you and coils up. Too late, the snake has bitten you.

Now compare this with the emotional brain response. A split-second before you even noticed the coil the limbic system has already decided that it is a suspicious object and, bypassing the thinking centres, has triggered an alarm reaction. You experience a shock of fear: your heart pumps wildly and your muscles tense. A split-second after that your emotional brain compares what is known about the 'stick' with other cellular memories, and reminds you what worked best in those situations (e.g. back away fast!).

The lesson here is that bodymind works many times faster than the conscious mind can. Thus, in order to keep up the thinking centres have to be quick off the mark. That requires it to be in a constant state of readiness. It helps if it is relatively clear of junk.

Here are some examples of emotional signals from cases seen in Reverse Therapy. It can be seen in each case that thinking mind is failing to respond quickly enough, despite the problem going on for several months, and more. As you read each example, I urge you to consider what a good response might have been.

Eileen – became tearful and anxious during arguments between her daughter, husband and grandson. She felt she got no respites from the family rows, that no one considered her own need for peace, and felt powerless to intervene. She hoped that the family would notice how distressed she became and cease arguing, but that strategy did not work. Gradually, as the rows continued, symptoms of acute pain in the neck, back and shoulders appeared.

Karen – heaviness, lethargy, and recurrent frustration appeared whenever her partner came home from work and 'dumped' his worries, problems and stress on her. Emotionally, she found it too much, but could not speak up in case her partner heard her as rejecting him. She hoped that, if she carried on supporting him long enough, he would grow up and stop dumping on her. But that did not work, either, and as time went on symptoms of nausea, muscle ache and brain fog appeared.

Steve – feelings of agitation, breathlessness, and heart flutter came on whenever he went into his teaching job, only to come up against another day of over-work. Covering for a sick colleague who was off work with 'stress', marking all the exam papers for the form, and covering his own teaching schedule. He thought that if he could only keep working hard enough, the work-load would stop piling up. At the same time he was angry that the school was not supporting him. But as time went on, with no resolution in sight, symptoms of fatigue, brain fog and muscle ache also appeared.

Possible responses:

Eileen: To lay down some boundaries, making her home off-limits to arguments. Another option is to absent herself from home when her daughter visits.

Karen: Ditto. To stop avoiding assertive communication, and speak up clearly about her needs around her partner.

Steve. He simply has to learn to say 'no', and refuse to cover for his colleague any more without support from the school. He might also want to have a closer look at his over-conscientious approach to work, and seek more life-style balance.

Notice that, in each case, Bodymind is producing emotions such as frustration, fear and anger, followed by low-grade symptoms of bodily distress. And in each case, the body waits patiently for the person to read the emotional state and break the impasse. Later, as the individual fails to adapt to the developing emergency, symptoms of Bodily Distress Syndrome emerge.

In a book I co-wrote in 2001, '*Communicate with Emotional Intelligence*' – we argued that there were two distinct strands of emotional intelligence. One is *interpersonal* intelligence: the ability to empathise and read other people's emotions. The other is *intrapersonal* intelligence: the ability to read one's own emotions and act appropriately. Almost by definition, sufferers from bodily distress have lost the capacity for intrapersonal intelligence. As a result they fail to respond to emotional imperatives.

We turn now, in the next chapter, to investigate the sources of bodily distress in more depth.

Key points in this Chapter

- Junkmind, based on Ego conditioning, is the source of worries, negative self-judgments, and alarmist thoughts
- The Ego is the person we think we ought to be. It is the source of many negative self-judgments

- Negative thoughts weaken resilience, and our ability to adapt to problems in the environment
- Bananas (compulsions) are a special case of ego conditioning
- Junkmind blocks and distorts access to emotional messages from Bodymind
- While the left brain grounds us in reality, the right brain is too easily distracted by Junkmind fantasies
- Exercising mind control, and disengaging from junkmind, is key to health and resilience

5

ABOUT BODILY DISTRESS

The symptoms of bodily distress

One problem when discussing conditions such as Chronic Fatigue Syndrome is knowing what to call them, while using a label that actually says something about the source, or cause, of the problem.

Consider what is wrong with this list of medical and psychological labels:

- Chronic Fatigue Syndrome. Means only that the patient has a lot of fatigue.
- Fibromyalgia Syndrome. Similarly – a person with inflammation of muscles.
- Adrenal Fatigue. An alternative label for CFS, but the problem is that the Adrenal glands are not actually 'exhausted' – just unresponsive to the overload of signals from the hypothalamus & pituitary glands.

- Medically unexplained illness. Says merely that medical doctors don't know what is wrong.
- Functional pain conditions. States that the pain has no known pathology.
- Stress-related illness. The term 'stress' is meaningless, as will be discussed later in this chapter.
- Hypochondria (Yes, some people still think these problems are 'all in the mind')
- M.E. – Myalgic Encephalomyelitis – means inflammation of the muscles and of the brain/spinal cord. While it is true that there is muscular inflammation in some cases, there is no evidence at all that inflammation of the brain or spinal cord is present.
- Post Viral Fatigue. Although many post-viral conditions exist, these are not the same as Chronic Fatigue Syndrome. Some researchers have argued that CFS is caused by a virus. One culprit used to be the Epstein-Barr virus, until it was shown that many sufferers do not have any Epstein-Barr antigens present. In fact no virus has ever been identified as common to all patients. Nor is the fatigue symptom equivalent to post-viral exhaustion, as I explain in the next paragraph.

Any viral infections which do occur in some sufferers of CFS are an effect, not the cause, of the disorder. As the HPA axis progressively over-works, immune system breakdown often occurs, leading to the entry of opportunistic viruses. The fact that this problem typically occurs early on in the condition has led to this confusion between effects and causes. But the fact that a viral infection is one of the first symptoms does not mean that it is a cause. If that kind of reasoning were true then having a high temperature would be the cause of the common cold.

In an earlier version of this book I called these conditions '*HPA Axis Disorder*', which description at least had the merit of pin-pointing the physical source of the symptoms. However, there is little point in using a label that isn't ever going to be in common use, so I have discarded it. Instead I have begun to use the phrase '*Bodily Distress Syndrome*' (BDS), a term invented by two Danish researchers a few years ago, and I hope this will catch on instead.

BDS is a new diagnostic category advocated by Fink and Schroder in 2010. They argue that Chronic Fatigue Syndrome, Fibromyalgia, Functional Pain, Irritable Bowel Syndrome and similar conditions are actually the same disorder. Using a check-list of common symptoms such as fatigue, nervous system arousal, gastro-intestinal problems, muscular pain, concentration problems, headache and dizziness (while ruling out all other potential causes known to medical science) they showed that over 90% on a sample of more than 900 patients reporting with CFS, Fibromyalgia, IBS, etc., fitted the criteria for Bodily Distress Syndrome. They state that BDS is *not* a psychiatric problem, and nor is it hypochondria. They do not state what the correct treatment should be for BDS but, given that medically treatable causes have been ruled out, it is fair to conclude that medical treatments are not envisaged.

One great advantage of the term *Bodily Distress Syndrome* is that it does point accurately to the fact that the body is in distress as a result of challenges from the environment, and a failure to resolve them. Prolonged exposure to such conditions creates a heavy load on the body and, over time, bodymind is forced to take emergency measures to deal with the crisis; measures which gradually result in symptom production.

These conditions are not new

In 1869 a condition was identified by George Beard, an American Neurologist, which he called 'Neurasthenia'. The symptoms classified for this illness were fatigue, headaches, muscle tremors, extreme sensitivity to noise and light, sleep disturbance, and poor concentration. Beard thought that this was a new disease, unknown before in human history.

A famous case of neurasthenia was that of Florence Nightingale, the nursing pioneer. She made her reputation during the Crimean War (1854-56) in which she went out to nurse British war casualties in traumatic conditions. The death rate from injuries was then 40%, a figure Florence, by means of superhuman work on sanitation, organisation of the hospitals, training of nurses, and intensive personal care of the soldiers, brought down to 2%. In 1856 she came home, but from then on was always ill with what was then a poorly understood condition. Her symptoms were fatigue, muscle weakness, headaches, nausea, breathlessness and heart palpitations – all now consistent with a diagnosis of Chronic Fatigue Syndrome (or Bodily Distress Syndrome). Despite her illness, Florence continued to over-work, this time campaigning to get the government to finance properly-built hospitals and staff them with trained nurses. She steadily became worse and was eventually bed-ridden for 6 years. Although there were improvements from time to time, and she lived to the age of 90, she never fully recovered.

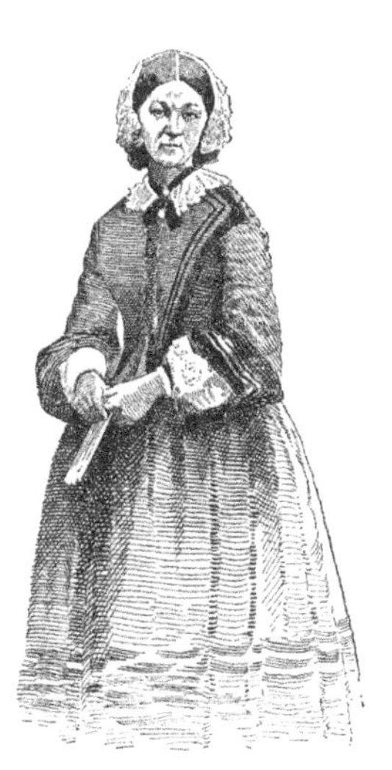

Florence Nightingale 1820-1910

Beard considered that the symptoms of neurasthenia were caused by too many demands on the nervous system. He pointed out that increasingly complex conditions of life in the big cities were creating ever more pressures on people. He argued that these pressures, if left unattended, gradually depleted the reserves of 'nervous energy' in people, leading to illness. A neurasthenic, he said, was a person who had used up these reserves and gone into 'nervous bankruptcy'. He prophesied that, as the industrialisation of the world proceeded, such cases would become more and more frequent. Indeed, there was an explosion of diagnosed cases throughout Europe in the last thirty years of the nineteenth century, just as there has been another explosion in cases of Chronic Fatigue and Fibromyalgia over the past 50 years or so.

Although neurasthenia, as a diagnostic category, was generally accepted there were no adequate explanations for why the symptoms appeared; nor was there a cure. The usual 'treatment' was seclusion and rest which, then as now, can only provide temporary relief for the symptoms.

Due to this lack of understanding, neurasthenia was too often confused with other conditions and, as a result, the term became over-used and was eventually dropped, as it became too vague a label to be useful. Also, Sigmund Freud, who treated several cases, regarded the condition as psychological and, because there were no tests for neurasthenia that could confirm a medical diagnosis his view became generally accepted. His opinion that neurasthenics actually suffered from hysteria (the majority being women) was also accepted, and many unfortunate women were committed to asylums for that reason. This mis-diagnosis of the problem, using different terms and labels, continues to this day, with most unfortunate effects.

Charles Darwin was another 19th century celebrity who may have had some form of Bodily Distress Syndrome. He suffered from a long list of symptoms which came and went over fifty years: fatigue, colitis, joint pain, numbness in the hands and feet, dizziness, heart palpitations, blurred vision, nausea and eczema. An exact diagnosis of his condition has never been conclusively established, but attempts have included Crohn's Disease, Chronic Fatigue Syndrome, Mitochondrial failure, Postural Orthostatic Tachycardia Syndrome (POTS), Post-Viral Illness, and Hypochondria (this last was what his friends thought he had).

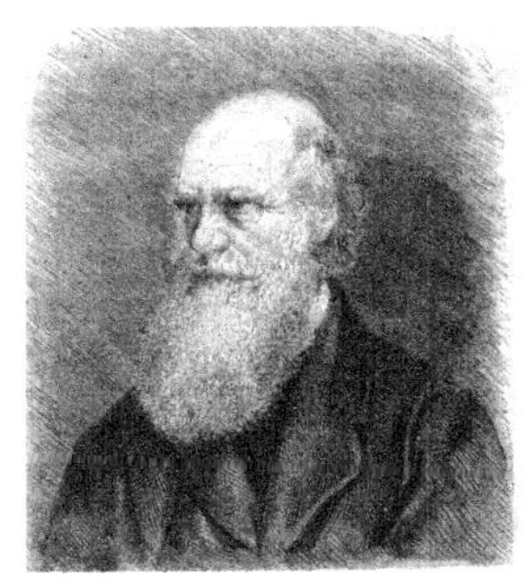

Charles Darwin 1809-1882

What is clear is that any type of 'stress' made Darwin's symptoms worse. Darwin was a chronic worrier who regularly overworked, bound to his desk, throughout his life. He also seems to have been emotionally constipated, and unaware of the influence of suppressed emotions on his physical state. He was distressed by criticism, and would run away and hide from any kind of conflict. He became upset when his observations failed to prove his own theories on evolution and he was unable to answer the objections of his critics (evolutionary changes were not finally explained until the 1950s, when DNA was discovered).

He experienced guilt because the controversy over his theories upset his church-going wife. Finally, he disliked publicity, and hated being in the public eye. Over the years he gradually became a recluse because, as he told his wife, he became 'over-excited' when with people, preferring to be on his own.

What is 'dis-ease'?

When the conscious mind splits from bodymind, and the two no longer work together in tandem, the resulting state of inner conflict is referred to as 'dis-ease'. In it we feel an inner tension, or discomfort, as blocked emotions and anxiety come to the boil, as if sitting on top of a pressure-cooker. It is this state of dis-ease which can, if left unattended, lead to the illnesses considered in this book.

In the 'dis-ease' state we are no longer comfortable with ourselves, with work, with home-life or in our relationships with other people. Dominated by the ego, we lose sight of who we really are, and we stop listening to our emotions. Instead we are racked by anxiety, forcing ourselves to stick with a life-style that no longer works.

Initially the state of dis-ease comes with uncomfortable feelings as bodymind draws our attention to the fact that we are out of balance. Deep down, we may know that something is wrong, but may not be able to put our finger on the problem or, if we do have an idea what it is, we may not know how to put things right.

In the early stages of dis-ease the answer to the problem may be quite simple. It could involve a talk with a partner, changing the schedule at work, or spending more time on things that are truly important to us. But if problems mount the state of dis-ease becomes more noticeable as Bodymind 'talks' to us more and more urgently. At this point we may become tense and anxious, worried and sleepless, more and more aware that we are becoming over-burdened. We may feel that we never have enough time to do all the things we think we have to do. As the state of dis-ease grows, junkmind becomes dominant and the thinking mind splits from bodymind. It stops doing its proper job of resolving emotions: identifying solutions, making decisions and taking action. This 'dis-ease' state is what many people refer to as the early stages of 'stress'.

The myth of stress

Some people mistakenly argue that Chronic Fatigue Syndrome and Fibromyalgia Syndrome are 'stress-related illnesses' as if, somehow, the word 'stress' explains things. There are two things wrong with this view. Firstly, the term 'stress' is meaningless and, secondly, the symptoms of CFS and Fibromyalgia are not directly caused by life challenges, 'stressful' or otherwise. Rather, they are the result of complex brain and endocrine reactions, designed to restore homeostasis.

The term 'stress' was first used by Hans Selye in the 1930s, and it was Selye who first identified bodily distress conditions and their sources. Working at the Prague General Hospital as a consultant physician, he noticed hundreds of patients with a variety of symptoms: fatigue, pain, digestive problems, heart palpitations, headaches and insomnia. Yet tests revealed little that was wrong. Like many outstanding scientists, he investigated his patients in closer detail, and looked for common patterns. What he discovered in nearly every case was that these patients reported a history of at least 2 years with significant life challenges: marital problems, financial difficulties, employment problems, housing and child-care issues being some amongst many. He argued these symptoms had emerged as the person had failed to adapt to life changes and felt overwhelmed by them. He called this condition '*General Adaptation Syndrome*' (GAS), and hypothesised that symptoms were created as a result of long-term changes to the nervous system triggered by life-problems. Later on, he identified that symptoms were produced through changed activity in the Hypothalamus-Pituitary-Adrenal glands (the HPA Axis).

Selye spent the rest of his life investigating GAS; its causes, origins, and potential cure. In 1936 he emigrated from Europe to Canada, where he resumed his research at the McGill University in Montreal. However, his native language was German and they now required him to teach and write in English. This caused some problems in the translation of his key ideas. When seeking to describe what I have called the 'dis-ease' state he coined the word 'stress', using an architectural metaphor in which buildings decay and crumble because of their exposure to ground forces, foul weather, and weaknesses in construction. The idea was that people fall victim to external circumstances and then fall apart. But this contradicted his real discovery, which was that medically unexplained illnesses arose from a failure to adapt to circumstances and that unresolved life problems created too much strain for the body to bear. The word 'stress' is possibly a mis-translation of the German word '*Bedrangnis*', which means 'distress'.

The term 'stress' cannot explain anything because it refers both to the cause of the problem and its effects. We can see this when we listen to people talking about it. One person will say '*I am stressed through work*' (cause of stress) while another will say '*I'm feeling stressed today*' (the effects of stress). Nor does the word explain why circumstances leave us feeling ill, or what exactly the stressed state really is. Anxiety? Burnout? Rage? Breakdown? Illness? The concept seems to mean any or all these things and is too vague to be of much use. Finally, the concept of stress overlooks individual differences. If you put two people in the same challenging job one person will thrive, while another will end up ill.

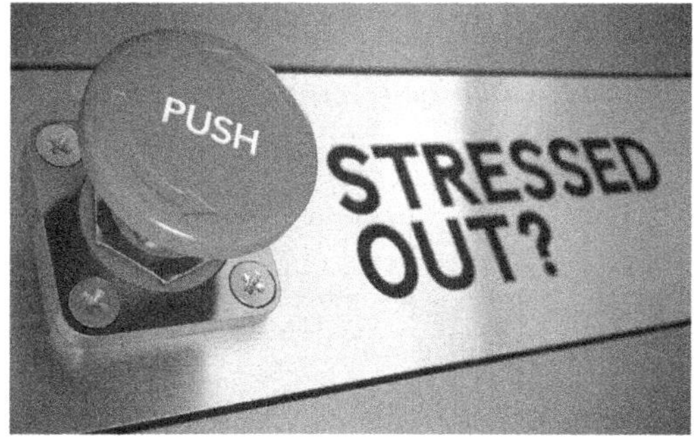

Cures for 'stress' are almost as vague as the problem

In other words, while the first employee is adaptable and resilient, the second job-taker is not. And it is these differences that we really want to know about. To be sure, some jobs (and some relationships) are abusive and exploitative and no sane person would want to stay in them for long. But the development of resilience in circumstances we *can* overcome is the key to staying healthy. Instead of using the word 'stress' when we think of *causes*, I recommend that we speak instead of life-challenges, overload and a loss of resilience. When we want to speak about the *effects* it is better to refer to anxiety, burnout, or bodily distress.

What is resilience?

Resilience is the ability to handle and overcome adversity. It has become the focus of study for researchers who seek to understand the difference between people who get 'stressed', and those who do not. Clearly, if we can identify the traits that resilient people have, then we can teach them to others. In that way cases of 'stress' would reduce, and so would the incidence of medically unexplained illnesses examined in this book.

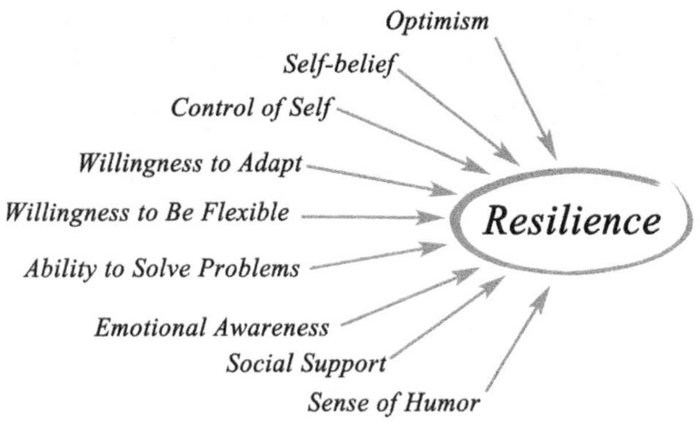
Optimism
Self-belief
Control of Self
Willingness to Adapt
Willingness to Be Flexible
Ability to Solve Problems
Emotional Awareness
Social Support
Sense of Humor
Resilience

Resilience - the ability to overcome adverse life-events - has been closely studied by Positive psychologists over the past twenty years.

As Hans Selye explained, these conditions arise from a failure to adapt to adverse life events. What then, enables resilient people to adapt where others do not? Below is a list compiled by me from my experience of working with such people over the years.

Self-aware. Attentive to their emotions, wishes and desires. Recognise when they are getting over-burdened.

Assertive. Able to articulate needs and emotions.

Good support networks. Gather around them friends, family and colleagues upon whom they can rely. In return they give support to others.

Problem-solvers. Focus on things they can influence, and on solutions rather than worries.

Know their limits. Are ready to say 'No' to unrealistic demands.

Maintain boundaries between self and others. Respecting others' needs and wishes, they also take care of their own.

Maintain balance. While attentive to their duties and obligations, resilient people are sure to take time out on their leisure pursuits, social networks, exercise routines, and self-improvement.

Practice mindfulness or other calming techniques. I am sure there must be resilient people out there who don't practice some form of meditation. I just haven't met one yet.

Low in anxiety. Staying out of junkmind, and exercising mind control over unwanted thoughts.

Alert readers may have noticed that many of the items on this list are the reverse of the traits Gabor Maté observed in people with auto-immune diseases. However, it is important to remember that those traits are reversible, and that resilience can be learned.

For more information on resilience I refer readers to a series of articles on the subject on my *Reverse Thinking* blog.

The onset of bodily distress

In what follows, I provide an overview of what happens to non-resilient people as the body approaches breakdown. It may be helpful to start with Selye's General Adaptation Syndrome, and it's three-stage development through an Alarm Stage, a Resistance Stage and an Exhaustion Stage.

During the alarm stage bodymind wakes up to the fact that the individual is coming under unsustainable pressure. As it takes action to stabilise the organism, low-level symptoms may appear as the HPA Axis swings into action.

In the resistance stage the body tries to adapt to the crisis ever more vigorously, but as pressures continue to grow the body struggles to maintain homeostasis (balance). The HPA Axis will be continually up-regulated. Towards the end of this stage symptoms may worsen significantly, and we may see initial immune system problems.

In the exhaustion stage the HPA Axis is no longer able to continue loading alarm signals on the adrenal glands which, due to overload, have become unresponsive. Symptoms become still more prolific, and immune system problems may deepen, leading to repeat viral infections, chemical sensitivities and other reactions.

In considering the mechanisms of bodily distress we will revisit the limbic system once more (I referred to it earlier in the chapter *About Bodymind*) focusing in more detail on three elements (see diagram, page 40):

- Hippocampus
- Amygdala
- Hypothalamus and the HPA Axis

Hippocampus. This is the place where cellular memories are stored and incoming information from the senses are routed through to it from the thalamus. Then matched with stored memories in the hippocampus. Information from these matches is passed along to the amygdala, and to the hypothalamus. Also onto the frontal lobes (front left on the diagram) for further assessment and decision-making. *As bodily distress progresses the hippocampus recognises a continuing stream of harmful experiences which are not being addressed.*

The amygdala is at the end of the hippocampus. Like the hippocampus itself, there are two of these, one on each side. The amygdala is the alarm bell in the brain. It helps to trigger emotion; angry bulls who have had the amygdala removed will become passive, docile and somewhat indifferent to their environment. Because of its strong links to the right frontal lobe, it is also the instrument for anxiety reactions. *As bodily distress progresses the amygdala is receiving a stream of signals from the hippocampus, which cause it to signal alarm reactions elsewhere in the brain, and to the nervous system. It also activates the Hypothalamus-Pituitary-Adrenal axis.*

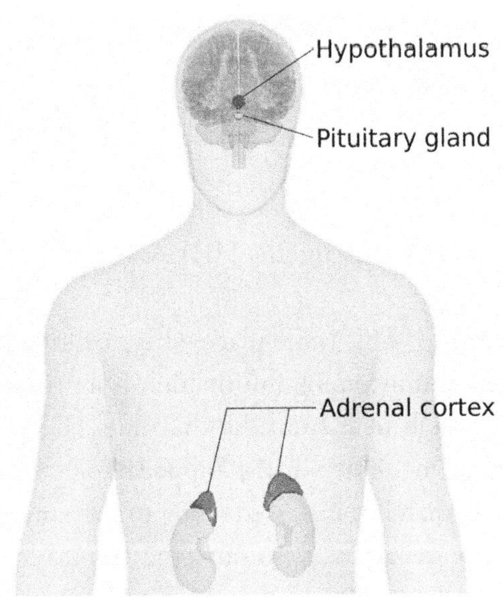

The Adrenal glands sit on top of the kidneys and contain over 60 messengers which impact on body function. The most important of these are adrenalin and noradrenalin (nervous system), dopamine (mood), and cortisol (immune system, metabolism and the rest-activity cycle)

The hypothalamus is, as was said before, the 'Master Controller' in the brain. It is crucial to the formation of both emotions and the symptoms of bodily distress. When alarm responses are received from the hippocampus, the amygdala and the frontal lobes, it releases a hormone to the pituitary gland below it, which then releases another hormone to the adrenal glands. Therefore, the HPA axis is at the core of the disorders described in this book.

Thereupon hormonal messengers are produced by the adrenal glands and sent on to the heart, lungs, liver, kidneys, pancreas, spleen, muscles, skin, gut, and the immune system. Specifically, the muscles work harder, the action of the gut slows down, and circulation changes so that blood is diverted to the major muscle groups. Activity in the immune system may be suppressed until the emergency has passed, because the immune system consumes a lot of resources which can be re-allocated to other functions. All these reactions result in symptoms of one sort or another.

The hypothalamus creates a variety of set-points to ensure that the organism is working at capacity. There are set-points for the immune system, hunger, thirst, pain, blood pressure, heart rate, digestion, temperature, breathing, energy regulation and sleep. During the 'exhaustion' stage these set points can no longer be maintained, as feedback mechanisms between the hypothalamus, pituitary and adrenal glands break down, and the hypothalamus gradually loses control over the body, which becomes still more distressed.

It is important to bear in mind at this point that symptoms such as pain and fatigue, headaches, 'brain fog', dizziness and abdominal discomfort are indirect communications to you from bodymind in which you are being invited to take urgent action to address the challenges with which you are faced. Resolving those challenges will return the HPA Axis to standby mode, and eventually to cessation of symptoms.

The simplified scheme below shows the complex mechanisms going on in the body:

LIMBIC SYSTEM
TRIGGERS
HYPOTHALAMUS
STIMULATES
PITUITARY GLAND
STIMULATES
ADRENAL GLANDS
CHANGE
MUSCLES – CIRCULATION – DIGESTION -
IMMUNE SYSTEM

Changes to the muscles are associated with fatigue, muscle pain and headaches. Those to circulation are associated with 'brain fog' and dizziness. Changes to digestion are associated with irritable bowel. Alterations in the immune system associate to infections, swollen glands, sore throat and feverishness.

In addition, the hypothalamus sensitises the optic nerve, which may give rise to light sensitivity and blurred vision.

The 'body clock' which exists inside the hypothalamus may also malfunction, which is one cause of sleep disturbance in these conditions. All the other symptoms of BDS can be explained by similar actions triggered in the limbic system and organised through the HPA Axis. One reason BDS is a multi-system disorder with a complex variety of symptoms is because these changes start at such a high level – in the brain itself. Yet the brain (limbic system) is responding to complex changes in the individual's external and internal environment.

The most significant problem in BDS, to my mind, is the one that affects the action of the muscles since it is from this that the two most significant symptoms – pain and fatigue – emerge. It is worth taking a closer look at this for a moment.

When the adrenal glands fire the muscles to work harder, the mitochondria inside the muscle fibres burn up large amounts of glucose and, as the glucose runs out, adenosine tri-phosphate (ATP), an enzyme which converts into an emergency source of energy, is used instead. It is this rapid burn-up of glucose and ATP which actually constitutes the 'fatigue' state. Meanwhile, the hard-worked muscle fibres become painful and inflamed, partly due to over-exertion, partly due to a buildup of lactic acid. It is important to realise that these symptoms are reversible once the ongoing emergency that gave rise to them has been addressed. This can be seen from the fact that the fatigue state can suddenly vanish, which puzzles sufferers who have been told it is 'exhaustion' or 'tiredness'. In fact, it is neither.

A guide to the symptoms of bodily distress syndrome

Bodily Distress Syndrome is a complex disorder and this account is simplified. The intention here is to help readers with these conditions understand how and why they occur. I hope these explanations will reduce the mystery surrounding these conditions. That done, fear over the symptoms can be dispelled.

Fatigue/Pain

I briefly explained these two core symptoms in the previous section when describing the action of the mitochondria in the muscles. Fatigue and pain are actually two sides of the same problem: overwork of the muscles.

Headaches

This is a special case of muscle pain. Here it refers to the scalp muscle tightening on the skull and creating pressure headaches.

Joint pain

Research has not shown that there is any clear-cut malfunction in the joints in either CFS or Fibromyalgia. It is therefore likely that the real problem lies in referred pain in the nerves that supply sensation to both the muscles and joints.

Poor concentration/short-term memory loss 'Brain fog')

This is likely to have several causes. One is a malfunction of the hippocampus which processes short-term memories. When sleep is disturbed, the hippocampus cannot clear daily memories, leading to overload. Reduced blood-flow to the brain, following on from changes in blood circulation to the muscles, impairs activity in the frontal lobes. Additionally, anxiety impairs short-term memory.

Blurred vision

In the general state of alarm, the hypothalamus fails to read light signals from the optic nerve efficiently.

Sleep disturbance

Due to problems reading optic nerve signals, the hypothalamus cannot process correct information concerning changes from light to dark, and from morning to night. This disrupts the internal body clock, and disturbs the sleep cycle. If anxiety is also present, then adrenalin releases will interrupt sleep.

Noise/Light sensitivity

In alarm mode, information from the senses is amplified by the Reticular Activating System in the brain. Sensations from light and noise are heightened, sometimes to a painful degree. Pain signals coming from the muscles are also raised, which adds to the fibromyalgia issue.

Temperature changes

Some clients complain of feeling too hot; a smaller number of feeling cold. While, in fact, their body temperature is normal. The reason for the problem lies in the fact that, as the hypothalamus is overloaded, it ceases to maintain its internal thermostat.

Viral and bacterial infections

Many people with CFS succumb to viral infections at the start of their illness. This viral problem is not the cause of the illness, but one of its effects. In the initial stages of the condition, the immune system overworks on producing antibodies to defend against infections. After a time, unable to keep up this kind of response, immunity is impaired, and opportunistic viruses enter the system, or are activated inside the body. An example of the latter type is the Epstein-Barr virus that causes Glandular Fever. In fact, most us carry this virus; but it never gets activated. With Bodily Distress Syndrome the Epstein-Barr virus - or other viruses - may be activated following breakdown in the immune system, leading to the mistaken view - based on confusing effects with causes - that viral problems cause Chronic Fatigue Syndrome.

Flu-like aches/Feverishness

This is also linked to over-activity of the Immune system. A common report I hear from my clients is that they feel as if they were always just about to 'come down' with an illness that never actually materialises, rather like the feeling one has in the first few hours of a flu infection. Aching/feverishness is caused by increased storage of antibodies in the lymph glands.

Swollen lymph glands/sore throat

In these disorders the Immune system is periodically up-regulated, which increases production of lymphatic fluid, swelling the lymph glands. Antibodies are diverted to the throat and create inflammation.

Dizziness (Orthostatic intolerance)

This is sourced by a combination of factors. Activation of the Sympathetic Nervous System causes reduced blood pressure, which is noticeable when the individual stands up too quickly. Reduced blood sugar (caused by burn-up of glucose in the muscles) also creates a light-headed feeling that adds to the problem. Finally, diversion of blood to the major muscles groups results in a 'pooling' effect in which blood supply to the head is decreased. Giving rise to dizziness.

Gut problems

When the body is in alarm mode, digestion slows and food is held in the stomach bowl rather than being released into the small intestine. This leads to increased gas and bloating, which is the source of stomach pain. If this start-stop mechanism occurs too often, it may lead to problems in the large intestine, and to irritable bowel. Increased stomach acid causes nausea.

Food and chemical sensitivities.

This is due to up-regulation in the immune system, which identifies as 'toxic' items which were before considered harmless.

How people get stuck in the illness loop

Anxiety over the symptoms, and the apparent disability which follows on from them, creates more symptoms as bodymind notices the person is worrying about the symptoms, rather than addressing their underlying message. It then triggers the HPA Axis to create more warning signals to the effect that anxiety, too, must be resolved.

Because sufferers so desperately want to get well, and be free of symptoms, they become very sensitive to the appearance of symptoms, frequently 'scanning' the body to establish whether symptoms have returned or got worse, becoming more and more anxious as they do so. After a while this checking response becomes a habit, thereby increasing worry and the associated compulsion to rest. When the 'radar station' notices this it triggers yet another alarm signal through the HPA Axis which creates fresh symptoms. Hence the illness loop:

Anxiety over symptoms > Increased symptoms > More Anxiety over symptoms > Reduced activity > More symptoms > More Anxiety etc.

This trap is in fact a 'negative feedback loop', and is the reason that some sufferers experience the same level of symptoms day after day in a wearying round of pain, fatigue and disability. It is also the reason so many people find recovery difficult. In the next chapter we will look at how Reverse Therapy resolves this loop.

Obstacles to recovery

Because of wrong information given to them by consultants who have failed to grasp the distinction between ordinary tiredness and the fatigue state, many sufferers believe they are 'exhausted', and that the solution is to rest. However, rest is not the solution. It is the thing to do if you are recovering from a virus, or from surgery, or if you have a wasting disease. It is not appropriate for Bodily Distress Syndrome.

Bodymind is looking for challenges to be overcome and emotional needs addressed – which won't happen if the person rests all day. Remember that the body will continue to 'turn up the volume' on symptoms as it notices that underlying emotions have been left unresolved. After too long a period of rest and withdrawal, frustration and boredom appear, as well as a loss of reward in daily activities. As these fresh issues are unaddressed, more alarm activity in the HPA Axis leads to renewed symptoms.

This last point is worth dwelling on, because it is quite subtle and gives rise to a lot of confusion. Say we have the fatigue symptom and then, one morning, we notice it has disappeared (because bodymind notices that emotional expression has improved, or because we have switched off from anxiety for a while). Not realising the true reason for this reduction we decide to take advantage of our good fortune, and go to work (or go shopping, visit friends, etc). We work for a few hours and all seems to go well, but then junkmind tells us we must not 'over-do' it and that we should go home and rest (here we might start 'scanning' the body for signs of returning symptoms, thus triggering anxiety and a rise in fatigue).

So we return home and go to bed for a while, or watch day-time TV, or trawl the internet for a few hours. Body-mind notices the reduction in significant activity, the slight increase in worry about the symptoms, and decreasing emotional satisfaction, and the HPA Axis raises symptoms to warn us to put an end to the rest period and go back to doing something more worthwhile. At this point junkmind concludes that we have made ourselves 'ill' again through doing too much that morning (or the day before). Anxiety increases and symptoms rise still more (this time in order to tell us to stop worrying) but junkmind screams at us not to try any more activities. Eventually we resolve to spend the next day in bed, hoping symptoms will once again mysteriously vanish.

Key points in this Chapter

- 'Bodily Distress Syndrome' has appeared under various labels over the past 150 years
- The concept of 'Stress' is not a helpful way of understanding the origin of bodily distress
- Loss of resilience is the real source of the disturbances that give rise to bodily distress
- Bodily Distress Syndrome appears gradually, in stages, as we fail to adapt to life challenges. From the initial 'dis-ease' state, through to emerging symptoms

- Symptoms of unexplained fatigue and pain, in particular, are warning signals which direct our attention to the need to address problems in the environment
- Misunderstandings about symptoms, combined with alarmist thinking, keeps us stuck in the illness loop. In which dread of the symptoms paradoxically results in fresh symptoms

6

ABOUT REVERSE THERAPY

What is Reverse therapy?

Reverse Therapy is a symptom-focused approach which teaches people how to work with bodymind, understand why the body has gone into alarm/distress mode, identify the specific triggers for the symptoms and to resolve symptoms by improving emotional expression, reducing anxiety/frustration, and improving life-style. Strictly speaking Reverse Therapy is not actually a therapy but an educational process. One reason we ask clients to read this book before making their first appointment is to assist that educational process in the making.

Principles of Reverse therapy

Here are some of the most important principles behind our work. Understanding them will help make it clearer to you how Reverse Therapy is effective in resolving the symptoms of Chronic Fatigue, Fibromyalgia and other types of bodily distress.

Reverse Therapy reverses attitudes to medically unexplained illness. We argue these conditions do not have a medical cure, although the symptoms are physically real. That these illnesses are not psychosomatic, but show physical distress. That we must reverse our thinking patterns and focus on the intelligence of the body, and the deeper reason for symptoms. We also reverse attitudes to the symptoms: instead of them as 'bad' we see them as signals that something is wrong with the client's way of being. We do not agree that fighting the symptoms is a good thing. That is rather like a driver noticing the oil warning light come on in the car, and deciding to rip out the light, instead of filling up the oil tank.

Symptoms are a form of intelligent communication. Symptoms result from bodymind activities that transfer information back and forth between the hypothalamus and the glands, the nervous system, the immune system, the muscles, skin and gut. These are really changes in particular types of information within the organism which we experience negatively only as long as we fail to understand that that these symptoms are alarm signals that call for change.

Attuning to Bodymind. We maintain a focus on bodymind communication in every session, and try to understand the distress behind the symptoms. Looking at situations in which symptoms have been produced and asking ourselves the question: 'If I were this person's body, what would I be trying to tell her about this situation?' Continually directing the client to pay attention to her symptoms as they come up, and get a feel for what bodymind is asking her to do. Some clients may find this difficult to do at first because they are trying to fight symptoms instead of understanding them. We reverse this, and help clients stay with the symptoms until their purpose becomes clear.

Mindfulness is an important tool in the recovery process. We teach mindfulness techniques, or encourage clients to practise their own preferred techniques, because mindfulness is a gateway through which the thinking mind can attune to bodymind. It is also helpful in reducing anxiety.

Reverse Therapy is an advisory process. We explain quite a lot about the Emotional Brain and the HPA Axis. Also, how and why symptoms are produced from them. By teaching them the facts about what is happening inside the body, and how people can get well, we dispel fear of the symptoms, replacing fear with hope.

Symptoms are signs of 'dis-ease'. Symptoms are not necessarily evidence of illness in the conventional sense. In the initial stages of bodily distress they are signs that the individual is undergoing environmental pressures, resulting in an imbalance between his personal needs and the demands placed on him. We encourage clients not to use terms like 'illness', 'sickness' or 'exhaustion' in describing their condition, as this obscures the fact that a deeper purpose lies behind the symptoms.

Bodymind naturally promotes self-healing. Left to itself, without interference from others, or from junkmind, bodymind uses first emotions, and then symptoms, to deliver its felt opinion about problems, prepare us for action, and show what those actions should be. Its primary purpose is self-protection and the restoration of balance. It also seeks to guide us towards adaptation to the environment. Once these purposes have been achieved, it spontaneously turns down activity in the HPA Axis, and symptoms can clear up.

Self-healing comes about through concluding emotional needs. Since symptoms are a communication of last resort that tell us that our emotional needs are not being met, concluding those same needs will enable Bodymind to switch off the symptoms. Emotional needs come in many forms, but all are based on being truly honest with ourselves: about times when we need help; when we need to speak up; when we need to let go; when we need to take time out for ourselves; when we need to do more to restore balance to our lives; and when we need to be authentic.

Realigning the Conscious Mind with Bodymind. Since 'dis-ease' comes about when there is a division between mind and body, bringing the two back into harmony with each other is integral to the recovery process. Junkmind may try to block emotions with rules that say that expressing them is 'bad', 'selfish' or 'impossible'. But when the thinking mind aligns with bodymind, it instead looks for ways to express emotions in ways that are practical, honest and reasonable.

The key to this approach is to understand the facts about symptom-messages. Many clients tell us that understanding the cause of the symptoms was the first step in their recovery. First, because it helped them lose their dread of the symptoms; second, knowing the cause also tells you what the solution is.

Using Empathy. Reverse Therapists use empathy and intuition in order to understand the unconscious intelligence of Bodymind. Empathy means putting oneself in someone else's position. In Reverse Therapy we identify with the client's body, developing a feel for what it is trying to express through the symptoms.

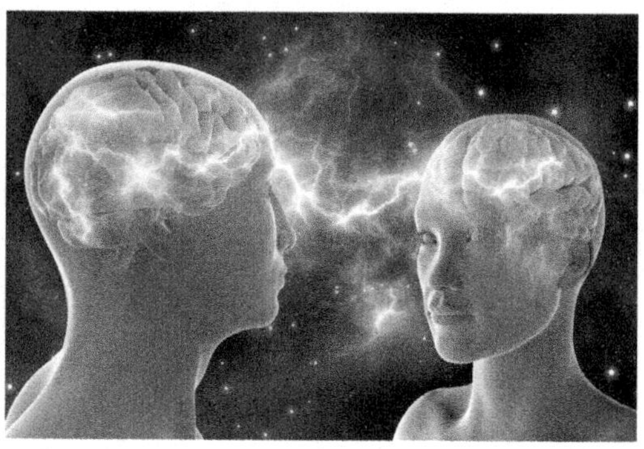

Empathy is not sympathy. It is the act through which we place ourselves in the other person's shoes. When we empathise, Mirror Neurons *in the brain fire, feeding us information about that person's emotional state, so that we can sense it for ourselves.*

Utilising intuition. Intuition is closely related to empathy, and refers to the ability to develop deep insights by noticing patterns in what people do. Intuition is usually 'unconscious' because we are not consciously aware of how we developed the insight. In fact, insight into another person's bodymind comes about because our own body is subtly picking up clues from that person's facial expressions, voice tones, gestures, posture and the emphasis on particular words. Bodymind absorbs and processes all this information with astonishing speed, translating it into feelings of one kind or another until we are in a position (with skill and practice) to translate these intuitions into words.

Reverse therapists are translators. Using empathy and intuition, we get a sense of what the body is trying to communicate through the symptoms. Once we have achieved that, we 'translate' the message into English (or the client's own language if we know it), writing it down on a card for easy reference.

Reverse Therapists are also coaches. Once we have understood the symptom-message we can begin the work of assisting our clients to make necessary changes. Significant changes might include:

- Channelling anger constructively
- Resolving conflict
- Asking for help
- Managing work, duties and obligations
- Asserting oneself

• Balancing what clients do for others, with what they do for themselves

• Disengaging from frustrating impasses

• Improving personal relationships (or ending toxic ones)

• Improving quality of life

• Switching off from negative thoughts

• Eliminating anxiety

• Learning to live in the present

Michael's case

Michael was twenty-two and had lived with Chronic Fatigue Syndrome for six years. During the second session we were exploring the first appearance of his symptoms at sixteen.

Michael recalled his parents had gone through a bitter divorce when he was thirteen and, against his wishes, he had been made to live with his father. Yet symptoms had not appeared until three years after that, and there was no obvious connection to the symptoms from that source.

Michael first noticed the symptoms while he was on a train journey to London, where he was due to spend Xmas with paternal relatives (he would rather have stayed in Manchester with his girlfriend). I asked him to recall sitting on the train as the symptoms came up.

He was struggling to understand what bodymind was trying to 'tell' him on the train through the symptoms when I put myself 'in' his body and sought to get a feel of what it was like to be on the train trying to communicate to Michael about that journey. What came up for me was that the train journey was a re-run of the aftermath of the divorce, with Michael cajoled into doing something he did not want to do (i.e., a cellular memory). I checked this insight with Michael, and asked him to sense his body with this communication in mind. Straight away he felt tearful and angry.

Following this discovery, we worked on a symptom message that urged him to be more assertive with others – putting his emotional needs into words they would find easy to hear and accept. I also encouraged him to allocate time with his family, friends and (current) girlfriend at his own choosing.

With practice on this problem, and additional work on some other issues, his symptoms cleared up over the next few weeks.

Applications of Reverse therapy

Reverse Therapy is not counselling or psychotherapy, although it has borrowed ideas and techniques from other therapies. It was designed to work with the conditions known as Chronic Fatigue Syndrome, Fibromyalgia, Adrenal Fatigue, Tension Myositis and Irritable Bowel Syndrome. However, it has also been successfully applied to Tension Headaches, Irritable Bowel Syndrome, Colitis, Eczema, and Psoriasis. With some modifications, it can also be adapted to resolving Auto-Immune diseases such as Rheumatoid Arthritis and Systemic Lupus. Finally, it can also work with Burnout Syndrome.

Reverse Therapy is not a 'cure' but a method through which self-healing can be achieved. The task of the practitioner is to lift the veil on the symptoms, and encourage the client to look within for the solutions which bodymind has already prepared.

Note: In my view, nearly all human beings experience bodily distress at one time or another. This may take a mild form such as an occasional pressure headache, or it may take a major form such as we see in chronic medically unexplained pain and fatigue. This occurs whenever we fall into the state of 'dis-ease' and neglect our emotional health. Reverse Therapists do not differ from the rest of humanity in this respect. The only difference is that we understand what our own symptom-messages might be, and can therefore do something about them.

Emotions and mindfulness: two more keys

A recurring theme in this book is that unresolved emotions are a key factor in Bodily Distress Syndrome. However, most unresolved emotions are really about unresolved problems with other people. Anger, frustration, sadness and fear have to do with problems created in our interactions with others, which Bodymind pushes us to address. The twin emotions of joy and boredom are related, respectively, to our success in creating personal fulfilment, or our failure. The emotion of disgust may be about animals and objects, as much as other people.

Emotions have manifold purposes:

- Maintaining boundaries between ourselves and others
- Self-assertion
- Seeking comfort and affection
- Moving away from, or towards people
- Disengagement from situations we cannot change
- Protection of self and others
- Sharing and support
- Getting help
- Diminishing threats
- Focusing on what excites us
- Pursuing self-fulfilment
- Maintaining a balanced life-style

The reader will recall Selye's discovery that non-specific illnesses arose from a failure to adapt. In the light of what we now know about the function of emotions, we can say that failing to adapt comes about because the person is unable, or unwilling, to listen to the body and exercise resilience. It is therefore a priority in Reverse Therapy that we restore that connection, and the insights that come with it. To assist our clients in achieving that connection on a consistent, daily basis we:

- Identify moments when bodymind was 'speaking' to them

- Teach them to stay in present moment awareness

- Decode the symptom-message using sensate focusing

A few people have little experience in accessing and relating to emotions, still less in uncovering the symptom-message. It is therefore useful to give them exercises which help them do this. One of these exercises is to identify an important decision from the past. For example: buying/renting a new home, accepting a job offer, or entering a new relationship. Then we ask questions like:

- What did you feel when considering that?

- Where is that feeling in your body?

- What is that feeling like?

- What choice was the emotion guiding you towards?

We can ask similar questions about other situations: meeting new people, choosing where to go on holiday, exploring a new venture, etc. The aim is to improve the client's ability to 'translate' feelings and emotions for themselves rather than rely on our doing it for them. If you are considering Reverse Therapy for yourself, try one of these exercises.

Exercises like these are easier to do if you practise mindfulness, and for that reason we supply free mindfulness tapes to our clients and ask them to listen to them for 20-30 minutes a day. There are many good mindfulness tapes and applications available free. For example, the mobile phone app *Insight Timer* has over 80,000 meditation tapes divided into sub-sections like Self-Esteem, Sleep, Work, Stress, and Anxiety. 99% of these are provided without charge.

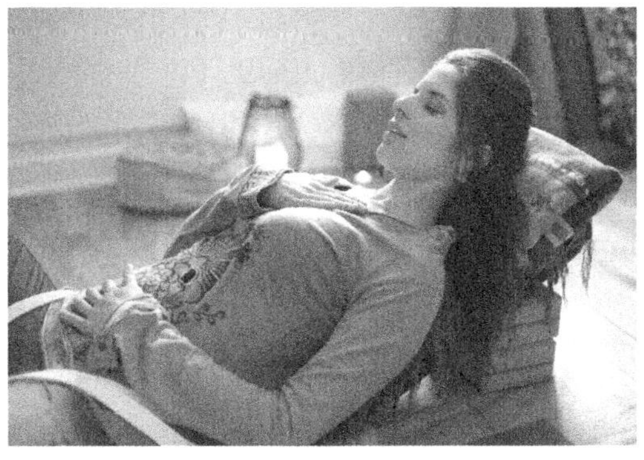

Mindfulness is a most effective way of disengaging from the overactive mind and developing present moment awareness.

A simpler alternative to mindfulness practice is Sensate Focusing, in which you hold your attention on the changing sensations of the body, especially the breath. Here is one approach:

• Select a quiet place in which you will not be disturbed.

• Sit in a comfortable chair, back straight and feet flat on the floor.

- Relax for a few moments and take a deep breath.

- Be aware of your feet pushing down on the floor.

- Be aware of your back resting on the back of the chair.

- Be aware of your hands resting on your lap.

- Now turn your attention to the movement of the chest and shoulders as you breathe in and out. Don't interfere with the breathing pattern – just train your awareness on it.

- Be aware of the air passing in and out of your nose and mouth.

- Now notice the time it takes for your body to breathe out, compared with the time it takes for your body to breathe in.

- Identify the slight space between the in-breath and the out-breath, in which your body pauses before moving the chest in/out again.

- Go 'into' that space between the breaths, right into the middle of your body.

- Hold your attention in that space for a minute or two.

- At this point you should notice a shift in awareness such that you feel more grounded in the body. The mind will also be relatively quiet.

Continue in this state of awareness for a few minutes more.

This is an exercise that you can practise as often as you like. It is good to use it when symptoms increase. This will enable you to get a better feel for what bodymind is trying to tell you about the situation you are in, free from the distractions of the thinking mind.

The Reverse therapy protocol

Once the client has a little skill in sensate focusing, we are then in a position to teach them the nine basic steps of Reverse Therapy, which are carried out whenever major symptoms, such as pain or fatigue increase. These are as follows:

IF symptoms increase

1. STOP what you are doing

2. MOVE AWAY from that environment

3. GO to a quiet place

4. FOCUS on the Body

5. CHECK the feelings (emotions) your body has now

6. REVIEW the situation

7. ASK: What did my body want me to do there?

8. GO BACK and do that

9. CHECK the effects of your actions on the symptoms

(Repeat steps if no result obtained).

We ask clients to perform these steps each time symptoms increase until this ritual becomes habitual to them. By degrees, clients gradually become so used to tuning into the body in order to sense the meaning of the symptom that this ritual becomes engrained.

These steps are not required when anxiety is present. If symptoms are increasing because the client is stuck in junkmind, a different approach is required. The reason for that is that, while emotions are communications from bodymind, anxiety is not.

Working with anxiety states

Recall that anxiety is not triggered by blocked emotion but through junkmind activity. Specifically, through worries (including worries about symptoms and 'illness'), catastrophic judgments, obsessions, 'bananas', perfectionism and guilt. As these disturbing thoughts come up from the right brain, the amygdala triggers the anxiety state. With anxiety, symptoms arise in order to guide us towards deleting the thoughts that trigger it. The symptom-message for anxiety states differs from the message that applies to blocked emotions, and so is the related protocol.

Protocol for symptoms triggered by Anxiety:

1. STOP what you are doing

2. MOVE AWAY from that environment

3. NOTICE the anxiety state, but do not associate with it

4. NOTICE that you were/are listening to junkmind thoughts, but do not dwell on them

5. REFOCUS your attention straight away on any activity that occupies the conscious mind in a pleasurable, calming, productive way.

7. CHECK that symptoms are also diminishing

8. KEEP REFOCUSING until symptoms diminish

If anxiety has become chronic, repeat practice in disengaging from alarming thoughts may be required. This, in turn, may require further tuition in mind control.

Uncovering the symptom triggers

There are three principal aims in the first session of Reverse Therapy:

1 To educate the client so that he or she clearly understands why the Body is producing symptoms

2 To investigate recent symptom episodes to uncover the symptom triggers.

3 To establish what exactly Bodymind is telling that client through his/her symptoms.

In order to complete the first aim, we go over some key points from the previous chapter, focusing specifically on how bodymind uses symptoms as warning signals. Also explaining that all symptoms are there to draw attention to something which is creating distress *in the moment.*

The reason I have italicised those last three words is because they carry a crucial point. That is because many people misinterpret the cause of the symptoms. Making the error that symptoms arise because of events in the past. For example:

• I am having symptoms now because someone upset me this morning

• I am having symptoms now because I did too much yesterday

• I am having symptoms now because I am still getting over my divorce last year

• I am having symptoms now because I had a tough childhood

As we saw earlier, emotions arise in the moment, and are about something that is happening in that instant. One thing that may seem strange to people who have not studied the subject is that bodymind does not have any conception of past and future; it operates only in the present. That is because it does not, like the thinking mind, employ concepts like time past and time future, but only in terms of cellular communications computed in a few tenths of a second in reaction to the present environment. To be sure, bodymind possesses cellular memories which preserve information about emotional experiences in the past. But it only uses those to gather a rough idea of what kind of experience you are having now. It is the thinking mind which contains episodic memories of events from the near or distant past.

Symptoms relate specifically to events that are happening right now. Having made this clear, we teach clients sensate focusing, and ask them to relive a symptom episode as if it were happening in the present moment. Focusing on what was happening around them, and what was seen, heard, thought and felt at the time.

If at the first attempt the client tries to interpret symptoms in terms of events that happened in the past, we gently redirect them to focus on what was happening in their experience a few moments before symptoms increased. We then identify the client's triggers.

In order to guide the client in identifying them, we explain that there are four main triggers:

1 Unexpressed emotions

2 Anxiety

3 Resentment/frustration

4 Loss of balance, variety and reward in daily activities

Let us probe each of these triggers in a little more depth.

Unexpressed emotions. Most emotions are commentaries on our relationships with people. Therefore, unspoken emotions largely relate to the demands other people place on us. And our needs, desires, hopes and wishes concerning those same people. I refer the reader to Chapter Three on this point. What bodymind requires is for us to express those needs as honestly as we can.

Anxiety. I have covered this subject in Chapter Four. When we pay too much attention to worries and other negative thoughts, bodymind pushes us to exit from junk-mind, and refocus as soon as possible.

Resentment. This one is based on junkmind demands of various kinds, relating to situations we cannot change. Demands that situations should be different from what they are, or things that have happened should not have happened. Note the use of 'must' and 'should' in some of these judgments. These demands can lead to intense frustration as bodymind pushes us to disengage from them. Here are some examples below:

I'll never get over what happened to me all those years ago.

I should not have to live with this.

People must not behave that way.

I'll never forgive what she said to me.

The symptoms are back again, dammit.

The answer is to let go of the ego's demands and bananas. Accepting that what has happened has happened, letting go of the past, and focusing on what we can do to improve our situation in the present moment. If we find it difficult to let go of painful experiences with other people, then we may need to go through a forgiveness process. Where frustration over symptoms are concerned, the imperative is to switch to an attitude of acceptance and curiosity, rather than resentment.

Loss of balance, variety and reward in daily activities. This is usually the result of misconceptions about fatigue and some of the other symptoms. In the belief that activities make the symptoms worse, sufferers reduce their involvement in everyday life. But doing this activates more symptoms, as bodymind calls for more stimulation, not less.

During the first session, we investigate a few recent symptom episodes to get an idea of the triggers that may be operating. In order to acquire fuller information, we ask clients to keep a journal recording episodes in between sessions. In this way we can check for more symptom triggers, and evolve the symptom message.

Uncovering the symptom message.

Once we have identified the symptom triggers, we can write out the symptom message. We use cards for this purpose, which clients keep with them for easy reference.

A symptom message spells out what it is that bodymind desires the person to do when faced with a symptom trigger. Since there are four main triggers there are, in general, four types of symptom-message. However, each message is tailored to the client. Using her own words and perceptions to make the message as clear as we can.

Another complication is that symptom-messages which relate to the expression of emotion will vary according to the emotion. I refer the reader to Chapter Three on this point, but here are some sample messages relating to three common emotions.

Anger. My symptoms are UP to tell me to STOP ignoring my anger and start speaking up about my rights NOW.

Fear. My symptoms are UP to tell me to STOP pretending things are OK and START asking for help NOW.

Frustration. My symptoms are UP to tell me to STOP going along with what other people want and take some time out for me NOW.

If we consider the four basic triggers, the varieties of emotion, and individual differences between people, then it is easy to see that no one person will have exactly the same symptom-message as another. Thus the formation of symptom messages is an art rather than a science. However, all messages have the same structure:

My symptoms are TELLING ME to STOP doing one thing and START doing something else NOW

Although that message is too general to be of much use in real life, the emphasis is always on changing what we are doing, thinking, or saying the moment symptoms increase.

Some clients will have more than one message. A common combination is to have one message for the expression of emotion, and another for the reduction of anxiety. In addition, most clients will require a daily message which calls for the restoration of balance, variety and reward in daily activities.

The long-term aim is to help clients establish their own symptom messages without the need for a practitioner. Reverse Therapy is a set of life skills which, once gained, enable the person to remain free from symptoms. Or, if they do return, then to address the symptom triggers, and follow bodymind's directives. Thereby restoring homeostasis and clearing symptoms once more.

Working with the symptom message

That we have established an accurate symptom-message does not mean that the client knows what to do about it. If the client does not have the necessary skills or experience, then we coach them in what to do.

Consider these symptom messages taken from cases I have seen over the past few weeks (writing in February 2021). Each relates to the four symptom triggers I described above.

My symptoms are UP to tell me to STOP ignoring my frustrations and SPEAK UP clearly about them NOW.

My symptoms are UP to tell me to STOP listening to Junkmind worries and REFOCUS on something better NOW.

My symptoms are UP to tell me to STOP chewing over things I can't change and FOCUS on what gives me satisfaction NOW.

My symptoms are there to REMIND me to do MORE activities that bring me balance, variety and reward TODAY.

The first message requires the client to practise assertiveness skills. Where assertiveness refers to the art of having tough conversations without giving way, or provoking confrontation. One excellent guide to these skills is in the book *Nonviolent Communication*, by Marshall B. Rosenberg, which is used in professional training courses all over the world.

In teaching clients these skills, we use a simple mnemonic to pick out the four key elements in assertive communication.

Even **C**od **N**eed **A**ir

Where **E** stands for Event, **C** stands for Consequence, **N** stands for Need, and **A** stands for Appreciation.

Starting with Appreciation, we acknowledge something about the other person's position. For example, "I can see that you are upset."

Then comes the Event we wish to discuss: "You're shouting at me."

Then the Consequence: "When you shout, it makes it difficult for us to talk."

Finally, the Need: "Please lower your voice."

The full message, which may need to be rehearsed for fluent delivery becomes:

> “John, I can see that you're upset. You're shouting at me. When you do that it makes it difficult for us to talk. Please lower your voice.

For more information on this approach please see the relevant articles on assertiveness training in my *Reverse Thinking* blog.

Clients who have never learnt how to assert themselves may require further coaching. Some will need help in establishing what they really want from the other person, others in finding the right words. Some will wish to learn to stay calm while they are delivering the message. However, assertive communication is a skill anyone can learn with practice.

If the symptom message relates to anxiety, or negative judgments (such as resentment) we teach clients how to switch off from junkmind. If that proves difficult, we show them how to resist and challenge negative thoughts, using cognitive therapy techniques. We also employ more elaborate techniques which have the power to dismantle the power of past conditioning. Finally, we recommend the use of mindfulness techniques daily (see above).

Work on the fourth symptom message, which relates to the restoration of balance, variety and reward, is described in the next section.

Rebuilding a healthy way of life

There are three paths to recovery in Reverse Therapy. One is to improve emotional release. The second is to refocus away from junkmind. While the third is to recreate a healthy life-style.

Bodymind doesn't just want us to be in tune with our emotional needs. It also desires us to live a full, active and expansive existence. If one word could sum this up, then it would be 'wholeness'. Interestingly, the Old English origin of the word 'healthy' – *hale*, also means 'whole', or well. Bodymind is not just concerned with survival, but also with our achieving the maximum of fulfilment. This is still more true when we are carrying responsibilities. Child care, work, financial obligations, running a home, parental care, paying taxes, supporting friends, household chores, dealing with troublesome people, overcoming illness – to name just a few. For most people, unless they have some long-term injury or disability, the body is fairly resilient. It can keep going long beyond a safe limit for short periods of time. But if we go on shouldering too many burdens for too long, without balancing them with restorative activities, then we are heading for burnout. Gradually, we are worn down by the treadmill and, before long, bodymind sends distress signals.

Regaining wholeness means we have to put more effort into balancing what we do for others, with what we do for ourselves (including those things we want to do with our families, friends and partners). One of the side issues with chronic fatigue is that people frequently withdraw from activities they used to enjoy. Instead, they settle down to an unsettled existence in which they don't actually do very much. Unfortunately, that impedes their chances of recovery.

Once our clients have understood the physiological basis for their condition, have lost their fear of the symptoms, and are taking steps to act on their main symptom-message, they can restore the balance, variety and enjoyment which is the final key to recovery. Often this step goes side by side with a gradual return to normal life. For those who have forgotten what a 'normal' life is the process will naturally be slower and more measured.

At this stage, which typically occurs during the second or third appointment, we draw up a list of activities designed to recreate an improved life-style using the following questions:

'What activities did you used to enjoy that you don't do now?'

'What activities do you still enjoy?'

'What activities have you always wanted to try?'

'What activities give you a natural high?'

We also distinguish between instant activities which clients can follow at any time (e.g. taking a walk, calling a friend, practicing mindfulness), activities which may take a little planning (visiting a friend, a weekend trip, going to see a movie) and activities that require long-term planning (taking a new course, returning to work, organising a summer holiday).

Every day the client selects a mix of activities which optimise balance, range, variety and enjoyment. We are careful to ensure that they balance the activities selected between work and play; doing things with others and spending time alone; between activities outside the home and those indoors. Since all of us have responsibilities, there will be chores to complete. We get the client to break up chores with break-out activities in order to maintain variety.

Based on the answers to the four questions given above, we help the client compile a list of things to do daily, and we review their record of daily activities at each appointment. In this respect, Reverse Therapy in its later stages is similar to Occupational Therapy.

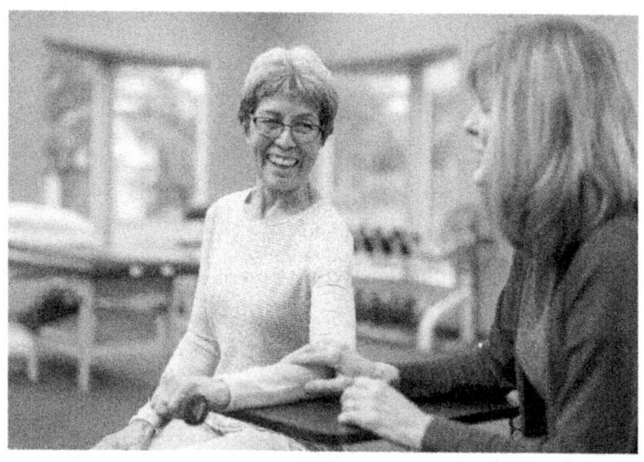

Occupational Therapists ask What matters to you?
Not: What is the matter with you?

Here are examples of two lists compiled by a client in Reverse Therapy. Notice that the first list is filled with activities, old and new, that she can do straight away, while the second list itemises activities that require preparation and planning.

Instant list

- Listening to music
- Dancing
- Singing
- Light reading
- Having a bath
- Calling a friend
- Self-Massaging (Hands and fingers)
- Walking
- Pilates exercises
- Watching something funny

Planned list

- Swimming
- Shopping with my daughter
- Visiting friends
- Art class
- Going to the cinema

- Going out for dinner
- Pilates group
- Having a massage

The endorphin factor

Both the 'Instant' list and the 'Planned' list shown above include activities likely to raise endorphin levels and it is now time to discuss these in relation to recovery.

The body produces at least 20 different types of endorphin, which are released mainly via the hypothalamus. They are neuro-peptides (the protein chains described before in Chapter Three) which descend through the spinal cord and the circulation of the blood. Endorphins are the body's natural opiates, and can be up to twenty times stronger than pain-killing tablets bought from a pharmacist. However, they are not just pain-killers.

Endorphins have several functions essential to health and recovery:

- Promoting calm
- Creating a natural 'high'
- Improving mood
- Reducing pain
- Enhancing immune system function
- Reducing blood pressure

- Counteracting high adrenalin levels
- Increasing energy

Activities known to boost endorphin levels include massage, meditation, yoga, dancing, movement (e.g. Tai Chi), singing, listening to music, breathing exercises, laughter, running, cycling, and swimming. Plus sex, dark chocolate and chilis. We should also include in this list affectionate times spent with friends and family.

One reason 'play' is so important is that taking time out just to have fun also raises endorphins. So is time spent fooling around, playing games and charades, as many children know. The ego rarely sees the point of (non-competitive) play, seeing it as a waste of time. But it is precisely because play is done for its own sake, without reference to rules and demands, that bodymind encourages it. By taking a break from 'bananas' and the urge to be always working or 'getting on' with things, we have the space to come back to ourselves, and live in the moment once more.

It has been shown that couples who are in a close, loving relationship are more likely to have elevated endorphin rates than people who are not. In fact, one important reason couples stay together is precisely because they give each other a regular 'fix' of endorphins. In Reverse Therapy we encourage clients to do as many things linked to endorphin release as they can manage, every day.

Finally, endorphins are energisers. Athletes who experience an endorphin rush while running report that they gain a second wind and, where before they felt unable to go on, now they can produce another burst of speed. The same occurs with people in recovery. The more they do this kind of thing, the more they find they can do, and the more their confidence in recovery rises. And so begins a virtuous cycle of increased activity, improved emotions, reduced symptoms, rising confidence, a return to work or community participation, and final restoration of health.

Misunderstandings about fatigue

This symptom - particularly in cases of Chronic Fatigue Syndrome - is the most poorly understood and many misconceptions abound. The most common of these is that fatigue is the same as tiredness. In fact, as I have shown, the fatigue state is in some respects a manic state in which the muscles are working furiously. The rapid burn-up of glucose and ATP that results creates the fatigue state. That can be reversed by attending to the symptom-message. Unfortunately, many people have been given the wrong advice by their consultants, and by self-styled 'Help Groups' who tell them they are in fact 'exhausted' and should rest as much as possible - or else to adopt a 'pacing and resting' approach.

To be sure, fatigue feels very similar to tiredness, and it is easy to mistake the two. Hence many clients are frightened to increase their activities as they believe, wrongly, that increased activity may lead to exhaustion.

Another confusion is that, for some people, symptoms appear to go up following activity. Sometimes this is based on a misunderstanding concerning time-lags, which I have explained before. For example, the client goes for a walk at 10 in the morning, with no fatigue arising then, but at 4 pm fatigue increases. The mistaken conclusion is that the walk six hours before is the cause of the fatigue that appears later. However, the two incidents are unrelated. As I explained above, increases in the fatigue symptom are always related to what is going on in the moment. Another example relates to increases in fatigue which occur at the end of the afternoon, or early in the evening. The simplistic conclusion is that activities that day have brought on the fatigue state. However, it is more likely that they are triggered by too little stimulation at that particular time, or by a deficit of balance and reward in that day's schedule.

A common reason symptoms may increase after activity (or even during it) has to do with anxiety. For example, the client visits the gym for an hour and fatigue increases while exercising. What is actually happening is that the client is worrying that exercise will make the symptoms worse. The symptom increases as anxiety increases, as bodymind signals it is time to switch off from junkmind, not to stop exercising.

Another reason for the increase in the fatigue state relates to confused ideas about rest. When fatigue is mistaken for 'tiredness' then rest seems the obvious solution. However, rest (especially that taken in bed) reduces balance, variety and reward. Resulting in more symptoms, not less. The same applies to the kind of 'rest' that involves watching daytime television, or playing around on computers for long periods of time.

Clients sometimes tell me that if they take a rest when they have fatigue, the symptom decreases. The reason that happens is not because rest works, but because taking time out from worries, demands and frustrations was the correct thing to do. But doing some other activity would have worked just as well. For that reason we distinguish between 'restful activities' and 'rest' where the latter really means doing very little. Restful activities that refocus the mind - such as mindfulness, listening to music or the radio, talking to friends, doing some gentle movements, or even having a bath will work just as well when the symptom-message is calling upon the client to slow down, take a break, or increase balance and variety.

In cases where clients have been ill for some time, their stamina and conditioning will be low, and they will require time to regain fitness. The solution in such cases is to set time limits on activities such as walking, running, or gym-work at first. Then gradually expanding the exercise range as stamina is restored.

Harriet's case (Part 2)

We met Harriet in the Introduction at the start of this book, and you may wish to refresh your memory about her case before reading this account of her recovery.

At the time I met Harriet she was mixing two or three days a week at her Law office with two or three days working from home, with her employer's permission. She experienced daily fatigue, brain fog, aches in her muscles and joints, and disturbed sleep. On investigation it emerged that the symptoms varied from one day to another with some 'good' days, and many 'bad' days. Interestingly, the 'good' days happened more often when she went to the office, while the 'bad' days occurred more frequently when working, or resting at home. Symptoms also ballooned when visiting or taking a telephone call from her mother.

I noticed Harriet looked tense and rather frightened, that she spoke rapidly and at length about her many problems, including her illness. While it is not always true that people who speak rapidly are dissociated from the body, it is a sign they may be anxious. That Harriet became visibly more anxious when discussing her symptoms, her work and career, and her problems with her mother, suggested that anxiety was indeed the most common trigger for her symptoms. That her symptoms were louder when she was working at home on her own during the week and at weekends confirmed this impression, as anxious people worry more when they are on their own or unoccupied. To paraphrase Parkinson's Law: worries expand according to the time available to think about them. And anxious people on their own too easily fall into rumination.

Other symptom-triggers were also present. Emotions of sadness and (disguised) anger were there: sadness over the ending of her relationship with James, and irritation with her mother's carping. Additionally, her quality of life was poor. From worry about the fatigue state she had stopped going out, exercising at the gym, going to the Yoga group she used to enjoy, meeting her friends or doing anything else at all apart from working and 'resting'.

Harriet was (or rather is) an intelligent person and had carefully read a previous edition of this book before coming to see me. Reading it had resonated with her as I described how worry and anxiety and blocked emotions linked to problematic relationships trigger the symptoms she had so far experienced. Prior to her first appointment, she had explored those connections for herself. She had also realised that she had to learn to take better care of herself before she could get well. All that she required from me was a treatment plan.

The first step was to change the work-rest cycle in which she was trapped. I went over the physical basis for the symptoms, emphasising that the fatigue state does not require rest, but change. We agreed she would spend less time indoors on her own; that she would go to the office three days a week rather than two, and on those days on which she was at home she would vary her routine with walks, phone conversations with friends, music (she was a trained pianist), and daily yoga practice.

The next step was to address her over-active thoughts and worries, and this was the target for her first symptom-message:

My symptoms are UP to tell me to STOP fretting and START focusing on something productive NOW

Mindfulness tapes were issued, and we also drew up an 'instant' list of activities that would refocus her mind: music, social contacts, piano playing, films, yoga exercises, etc. I also asked her to write down any persistent worries for further work on the next session.

In an email I received the day before our next appointment Harriet told me there had been some improvement and she had experienced two afternoons with no symptoms at all - once at work and also on a Saturday afternoon which she spent with two girlfriends.

We ask all clients in Reverse Therapy to keep a journal tracking the rise and fall of symptoms and the associated triggers. Looking at this at the start of the next session, the picture became clearer still. Symptoms increased when she worried, and also during phone calls from her mother. She worried about the future, about whether she could manage her work-load, and that she might lose her job. Although there were also unresolved emotional problems with her mother, I felt we could not work on this issue until the fog of over-thinking, worry and obsession had been cleared.

There were some underlying concerns underpinning two major worries which also needed attention:

Concerns about her work-load. As is common in people with Harriet's over-conscientious approach to life, she took on too much work and spent too long on perfecting the work, when the job had already been completed to a satisfactory standard. She no longer believed that fatigue and pain stopped her working, as she had demonstrated to herself that this was not so: it was anxiety that triggered these symptoms, not work. Harriet told me that her line manager had several times asked her to delegate work to other members of the team whenever she wanted. But she did not do that too often, as she thought people would judge she was incapable. In fact, this was not true: they considered her a valuable member of the team. She therefore agreed to hand over a new case that had been passed to her for attention, and to ask another colleague to undertake some research on her behalf for two other cases that she was preparing.

Coping with visits and phone calls from her mother. I gathered that Harriet's mother would call her for over an hour at a time, mostly talking about herself and her own problems, pausing from time to time to pass on unsolicited opinions to Harriet about what she should do with her life. Personal visits followed much the same pattern. Harriet felt overwhelmed by the sheer volume of talk. Although there were deeper, emotional issues to deal with, the priority was to develop new strategies for managing calls and visits. We agreed Harriet would limit calls to no more than 20 minutes, explaining that she had other appointments to go to, or work to finish. I also suggested that Harriet visit her mother, rather than the other way around, as that would give her more freedom to come and go, and to put an end to the visit at a time of her own choosing. I advised Harriet that keeping boundaries in place and being firm on this point would take much practice, as it was something she had never done with her mother before.

On this and subsequent appointments, I taught Harriet a variety of methods throughout which she could disengage from junkmind content. Some were based on mindfulness, others were mind control techniques, while others targeted the thoughts themselves, demolishing them with facts, logic and fresh perspectives. I will not describe these techniques here as that would take up too much space, but many of them are described on my *Reverse Thinking* blog. Suffice to say, the result of all these techniques is to change one's attitude to junkmind thoughts until we reduce them to random noise: like the static you might hear coming up during a radio program.

After four sessions Harriet had reduced the time wasted on junkmind, and her symptom episodes had reduced by over half. But the next four sessions were far harder, as we addressed her relationship with her mother. When Harriet attuned to her body's feelings about her mother, she encountered fear that meeting her mother might overwhelm her. Also, there was a fear of being abandoned, which was linked to the sadness she felt over the recent ending of her relationship with James. The third emotion was anger at how her mother constantly invaded her life, cajoling and hectoring her by turns. Each of these emotions, and their associated action-cycles, were addressed in turn, beginning with her fear.

The help and support she required were already available to her through our professional relationship as well as from her friends. I also discovered that Harriet had an aunt, her mother's younger sister, whom she knew had similar concerns about her mother's attitude, and who was kind and attentive to Harriet. This aunt lived in York, but Harriet travelled up, and spent a long weekend with her and her family. During conversations with her aunt Harriet realised that her mother was a troubled person: lonely, self-doubting and anxious herself. That she, too, had suffered over the break-up of her own marriage, and her worries about her daughters, although she had an unhelpful way of expressing them, masked a genuine concern for their welfare. Her excessively high standards for Harriet and her sister were propelled by the hope that her two daughters would have a better life than she'd had herself.

Talking over this insight, I suggested to Harriet that she should express appreciation for her mother's efforts, while politely telling her she was old enough to make her own decisions now and could be left to get on with making them. We practiced different ways of putting this message into words using the assertiveness technique described earlier, and Harriet agreed to speak to her mother.

Sadly, this did not go well and Harriet's mother interpreted her well-meant efforts as a rejection and refused to speak to her for some months. Although this put a stop to her phone calls and visits for a while, Harriet was naturally upset. Even so, Harriet's symptoms reduced still more significantly. Five months after first seeing me she experienced only occasional fatigue and pain, which she had now learnt to see came up when she was worrying, or getting over-conscientious. Disengaging from junkmind, slowing down, and delegating work, would quickly pacify those.

A few months after her last appointment she emailed to tell me she and her mother were now talking and meeting again and, although their relationship was a little strained, her mother had told her that she thought Harriet was 'grown-up' now and wouldn't be needing much help from her anymore. The fraught phone calls had also ceased.

Preparing for your first session

If you are thinking of coming for Reverse Therapy yourself, there are several things you can do to prepare for your first session.

Reading this book will, I hope, have given you a clearer idea of how the approach works. You can also read the case studies on the Reverse Therapy website for more real-life examples of recovery from Fibromyalgia and Chronic Fatigue. Finally, there are three video interviews with past clients of Reverse Therapy on our YouTube channel.

Practice doing the sensate focusing activity described earlier in this chapter, or listen to one of the mindfulness tapes recommended. If you already practice yoga, tai chi, the Feldenkrais method, or pilates exercises, or anything similar, then increase the time you spend on those methods. Try to get a greater feel for how your body might use symptoms to warn, guide, and protect you while practicing one of these disciplines.

After you have read this book, consider your ideas about 'health'. What does that word mean to you? When have you been at your healthiest and what practices were you following at that time? More importantly, what will you be doing when you get well and what healthy practices will you be following that you aren't following now?

Next, consider the history of your symptoms and address the following questions (it can help to write the answers down):

• What was happening in your life in the weeks and months just before symptoms first appeared?

• What challenges/problems were you dealing with at that time?

• What emotions can you recall from that time? What do you feel bodymind would have liked you to do about them?

• What 'bananas' and worries and other negative judgments were you listening to at that time?

• What emotions were you not having that others might have expected you to have? For example, if you were being swamped with unfair demands from other people and you were not getting angry, it may well be that junkmind was blocking the anger, and bodymind wanted you to reconnect.

• How good was your work-life balance? How much time were you devoting to social activities, leisure pursuits, and doing other things you enjoyed? Might your body have felt that you were spending too little time on these things, and too much time attending to duties and obligations?

• What else might your body have been trying to encourage you to do?

Now ask the same questions just given in relation to the past month.

• Are the same problems and challenges still present? Or are they now different?

• Are you less active now than you were at the time symptoms first appeared?

• Are you more anxious now (about symptoms) than you were before?

• What triggers for the symptoms are present on your 'bad' days?

• Now have a look at the opposite question: what is going on during your 'good' days that might give some clues to reducing symptoms?

Have you had any mornings, afternoons, or days recently when symptoms disappeared or reduced significantly? What was happening at those times? Be careful to note whether any of the following may have applied to you:

• Engaging in conversations with partners, friends and family and telling them how you feel about things?

• Engaging in rewarding pursuits?

• Working purposefully?

• Maintaining balance and variety that day?

• Speaking up honestly to people?

• Taking more time out for you?

• Doing things that improved your confidence?

• Asking for support from others?

• Switching off from worries and other negative thoughts, and focusing attention elsewhere?

(Note: if symptoms – especially fatigue – are pretty much on the same level day after day, this is most likely due to stagnation. Bodymind will use persistent, daytime symptoms to encourage you to move out of the 'illness loop'. Engaging in a varied, more active lifestyle, taking small steps each day towards doing so).

Now consider what wellness means to you. If it means simply going back to the routines that existed before you developed symptoms, you may need to reconsider. Your recovery will ultimately depend on your adoption of a lifestyle that supports wholeness. This may mean balancing work with leisure; creating more time to do your own thing; being more emotionally honest with other people; saying 'no' more often; and, above all, following activities that bring you inner peace, love, growth and personal fulfilment. It may mean taking a new direction in life. Above all, your return to health means learning how to be true to yourself.

What do you truly love to do? What is it that most expresses the real you? Your answers don't have to be 'big' answers. The real you might yearn to spend quiet times with your family, get back to gardening, or sharing a meal with your friends. Answers might also include taking a fresh course of study, moving to a different part of the country, or changing jobs. Whatever the answers are, finding out what matters to you will be an important part of your recovery.

If, having read this book, you are still not convinced you can recover, then look harder at the negative effect junk-mind may have on you. Maybe your mind is filled with the negative ideas, judgments and hopelessness that you acquired from people with the same illness, or from the failure of other treatment approaches. Be ready to reverse out of those ideas and consider a new perspective. Notice how junkmind keeps you trapped in the past, or in a present-day cycle of negativity, worry and 'disaster-movies' based on those poor experiences. Remind yourself that you did not understand the symptoms then, and that this book has given you fresh understanding. Do small things to break out of the cycle, focusing on things you enjoy, or activities that provide a sense of achievement. As your symptoms fade, your confidence will grow.

Wishing you a swift recovery to health through the symptom path to enlightenment!

Key points in this Chapter

- Reverse Therapy is an educational process which teaches people to understand and work with bodily distress
- Reverse Therapy is a symptom-focused approach which addresses the deeper purpose behind the symptoms of Chronic Fatigue and Fibromyalgia
- The initial session focuses mainly on uncovering the symptom-triggers, and their associated symptom-message
- Reverse therapists employ empathy and intuition to uncover the symptom message, then coach clients to take effective action
- Mindfulness practice is key to this approach
- Emotional resolution, disengagement from anxiety, releasing frustrations, and restoring balance, variety and reward to daily life are the basis for most symptom messages

7

APPENDIX 1 - SELECT BIBLIOGRAPHY

William Bloom. *The Endorphin Effect.* 2001.

Anna Budtz-Lilly et. al. *Bodily Distress Syndrome: A new diagnosis for functional disorders in primary care?* 2015.

Don Colbert. *Deadly Emotions.* 2003.

William Collinge. *Recovering from M.E.* 1993.

Antonio Damasio. *Descartes' Error.* 1994.

Antonio Damasio. *The Feeling of What Happens.* 1999.

Richard Davidson and Sharon Begley. *The Emotional Life of Your Brain.* 2013.

Henry Dreher. *Mind-Body Unity.* 2003.

Ken Dychtwald. *Bodymind.* 1977.

Barry Gibb. *Rough Guide to the Brain.* 2007.

John Eaton. Reverse Thinking Blog at www.reversethinking.co.uk

John Eaton and Roy Johnson. *Communicate with Emotional Intelligence*. 2001.

Milton Erickson. *Collected Papers, Volumes I-IV*. 1980.

Eugene Gendlin. *Focusing*. 2003.

Daniel Goleman. *Emotional Intelligence*. 1996.

David Jameson. *Mind-Body Health and Stress Tolerance*. 2003.

Byron Katie. *Loving What Is*. 2002.

Joseph LeDoux. *The Emotional Brain*. 1999.

Joseph LeDoux. *The Synaptic Self*. 2002.

Paul Martin. *The Sickening Mind*. 1997.

Gabor Maté. *When the Body Says No*. 2003.

Dan Neuffer. *CFS Unravelled*. 2013

W.H. O'Hanlon & A.L. Hexum. *An Uncommon Casebook*. 1990.

Tim Parks. *Teach Us To Sit Still*. 2010.

Candace Pert. *Molecules of Emotion*. 1997.

Steven R. Pliszka. *Neuroscience for the Mental Health Clinician*. 2003.

Marshall B. Rosenberg. *Nonviolent communication.* 2015.

Ernest Rossi. *The Psychobiology of Mind-Body Healing.* 1986.

Ernest Rossi. *The Symptom Path to Enlightenment.* 1996.

John E. Sarno. *The Mindbody Prescription.* 1998.

John E. Sarno. *The Divided Mind.* 2006.

Hans Selye. *The Stress of Life.* 1978.

Esther Sternberg & Philip Gold. *The Mind-Body Interaction in Disease.* (Scientific American – Special Issue). 1997.

Liz Tucker. *When You Want to Say Yes But Your Body Says No.* 2003.

Margaret Wehrender and Steven M. Prinz. *The Anxious Brain.* 2007.

8

APPENDIX 2 - SCIENTIFIC PAPERS

Selected papers which evidence the involvement of the HPA Axis in Chronic Fatigue Syndrome, Fibromyalgia and other conditions related to bodily distress.

Evidence for and pathophysiologic implications of hypothalamic-pituitary-adrenal axis dysregulation in fibromyalgia and chronic fatigue syndrome. Demitrack, M.A. and Crofford, L.J. Annals of the New York Academy of Sciences, May 1998

Function of the hypothalamic-pituitary-adrenal axis in patients with fibromyalgia and low back pain. Griep E.N, Boersma J.W., Lentjes E.G., Prins A.P., van der Korst J.K., de Kloet E.R. Journal Rheumatology. 1998 July; 25(7): 1374-81

The role of the hypothalamic–pituitary–adrenal axis in rheumatoid arthritis. Agnes M., Eijsbouts M., & Murphy P. Best Practice in Research Clinical Rheumatology Volume 13, Issue 4 , December 1999, Pages 599-613

Hypothalamic involvement in chronic migraine. Peres M., Sanchez del Rio' M, Seabra' M., Tufik S., Abucham' J., Cipolla-Neto' J., Silberstein' S., Zukerman, E. Journal of Neurological and Neurosurgical Psychiatry 2001;71:747-751

Basic pathophysiologic mechanisms in irritable bowel syndrome. Emeran A. Mayer, Bruce D. Naliboff, Lin Chang. Digestive Diseases 2001;19:212-218

Hypothalamic-pituitary-adrenal axis reactivity in chronic fatigue syndrome and health under psychological, physiological, and pharmacological stimulation. Gaab J., Hüster D., Peisen R., Engert V., Heitz V., Schad T., Schürmeyer T.H., Ehlert U. Psychosomatic Medicine: November-December 2002. Volume 64, Issue 6: 951-962

The HPA axis and the genesis of chronic fatigue syndrome. Cleare A. J. Trends in Endocrinology and Metabolism. Volume 15, Issue 2, 2004: 55-59

Neuroendocrine responses to psychological stress in patients with myofascial pain. Yoshihara T., Shigeta K., Hasegawa H., Ishitani N., Masumoto Y., Yamasaki Y., Journal of Orofacial Pain. 2005;19(3):202-8.

Chronic Fatigue Syndrome. Prins J.B., van der Meer J.W., Bleijenberg, G. Lancet 2006; 367:346–355

Hypothalamic-pituitary-adrenal-axis function in chronic fatigue syndrome. Van Den Eede, F., Moorkens G., Van Houdenhove B., et al: Neuropsychobiology 2007; 55:112–120

Hypothalamic-pituitary-adrenal axis dysfunction in chronic fatigue syndrome. Papadopoulos A.S., Cleare A.J., Nat. Rev. Endocrinol. 2011 Sep 27;8(1):22-32

A review of hypothalamic-pituitary-adrenal axis function in chronic fatigue syndrome. Tomas C., Newton J., Watson S. ISRN Neuroscience (Online) 2013.

Made in the USA
Las Vegas, NV
26 April 2021

22081754R00108